GATHERING ROSES

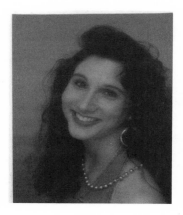

BY ELLEN WEISBERG

"One million people commit suic..."
The World Health Organiza...

All rights reserved, no part of this publication may be
reproduced by any means, electronic, mechanical
photocopying, documentary, film or in any other format
without prior written permission of the publisher.

Published by
Chipmunkapublishing
PO Box 6872
Brentwood
Essex CM13 1ZT
United Kingdom

Copyright © Ellen Weisberg 2007

http://www.chipmunkapublishing.com

To my husband Ken, with love

In memory of my friend, John

Thank you to Frank Williams, Deb Daigle, and Kenny Colville for their invaluable contributions to "Gathering Roses," and for all of their love, friendship, and inspiration

Proceeds from the purchase of "Gathering Roses" are to go to the American Heart Association

Prologue

Lori curled her body into a fetal position on Nick's bed and rested her head on his shoulder. Their dance was nearing its end as he lay next to her, only a few months away from leaving her for good. As her fingertips moved from the coarse, dark hairs on his chest down to his stomach, she thought about the games, the teases, the chases... She lay there with his arm wrapped around her, his hand gently massaging the small of her back. She thought about all of the things that had made him seem like so little to her; the things that made her feel like nothing to him. She moved her mouth closer to his, wanting to narrow the distance that she had been sensing for so long. He pressed his lips against hers and began passionately kissing her. He lifted her hand off of his stomach and rested it back on his chest. She could feel his heart beating fast and hard.

"See?" he said. "It's working *now*." He quietly laughed.

The games, the teases, the chases. The emptiness. The distance. She stared into Nick's dark blue eyes and saw the reflection of someone who could finally see that there really was something. There was something to everything that Lori had believed held no meaning. There was something to him. There was something to her, and there was something to what they both were to each other. There was something to *life*. And perhaps, at long last, it was time for Lori to start finally living it.

***

Chapter 1

Happiness is nothing more than good health and a bad memory
Albert Schweitzer (1875-1965)

The dawn sky was just starting to lift from solid black to a soft shade of blue when Lori pulled her car into the station's lot. She stepped onto the pavement and peered at the disheveled, turn-of-the-century building, with its darkness and unsettling stillness. There was one window ajar on the second level, through which Lori could see a dim, red light and hear a faint rhythm. She walked through the front entrance and dialed a three-digit code listed on the cardboard-thin wall for the radio station's control room. A loud buzzer sounded shortly afterward and unlocked an inner glass door.

Lori knew where the control room was from the few times she had observed the station's program director operating the mixing board. She quickly ascended a long flight of carpeted stairs leading up to the room she had seen from outside in the parking lot. She slowly opened the door.

"Hey, there," Nick said, cheerily. He glanced up at her for only a brief second before turning his attention back to the knobs and levers of the mixing board. "Take a seat. Lori, right?"

"Yes."

"You can watch me for a while, okay?"

"Okay."

"This is a pretty easy one. It's a gardening show. No special liners or sound effects. Ya just let 'em talk."

Lori placed her purse next to an open carton of yogurt on a shelf, and then quietly sat down on a metal chair and positioned it to face him. She tried absorbing the pattern of his hand movements as they glided from one end of the board to the other, but he was going far too quickly for her. She reminded herself that this was just a college internship, and that she'd get credit for doing it no matter how bad she was at it.

She blankly stared at a rose tattoo on Nick's thin, muscular upper arm. Dressed in a concert t-shirt and baggy polyester pants, he had dark, spiky hair cut close to his head and a frizzy pony tail jutting out the back. Lori's own hair was unwashed and lifted off her forehead with a brown, plastic headband. Because she had been running late, she was wearing the same gray sweatshirt with matching sweatpants that she had slept in the night before. Ordinarily, she would have been self-conscious about her appearance, but Nick didn't seem to be paying much attention to her. He was focused mainly on overseeing the mixing board in front of him.

"So how long have you been here for?" Lori asked.

"Oh, about seven months." He placed one hand on his hip and kept the other pressed against the gain pot, keeping a close eye on the levels of the VU meter. Soft, muffled voices were coming through the audio board and making the meter rock steadily back and forth.

The room suddenly got very quiet. It was too early on a Sunday morning for there to be much of anything in the way of background noise, such as the bustling kind you would hear on a weekday afternoon with cars and trucks whirring past on a nearby roadway. With the eerie silence penetrating the dust-filled air of the control room like a sharpened sword, Lori struggled to keep the room filled with sound. Any kind of sound. "So what…" She moved her body closer to the edge of her chair. "What were you doing before?"

"Before when?" he asked.

"Before you started working here."

"I used to follow the Grateful Dead," he said, stretching his arms out to both sides and opening his mouth wide in a yawn. "I uh... did a lot of traveling. Got to see all sorts of places, meet all kinds of people, experience..." He stopped.

"What?"

"Oh, you know..." He chuckled and raised his eyebrows high into his forehead. "Experience... all sorts of ... experiences." The chuckling turned into laughter.

Lori sat quietly and looked at him for a moment. "What uh..." She noticed a fly had landed on her wrist. Its legs were tickling her. "What did you do for money?" She lifted her arm up and shook the fly loose.

"Oh, you know," he said.

Lori continued looking at him.

"This and that."

The fly landed on a black gain pot at the edge of the mixing board. Nick shooed it away with his hand. "I got by," he said. "It was just for a few years. Decided to give it a break on my twenty-first birthday this past April." He looked at Lori, as though waiting for a response. She stared back at him, not knowing what he expected her to say.

"Do you believe me? Or are you starin' at all the little gray hairs on my head and thinkin' to yourself, 'there's no way...'"

"No. I believe you. I can't really see the gray hairs," she said.

"They're from all the drugs I did." He started to laugh.

"Ah," she said. She didn't know whether to stay straight-faced or smile. Was he joking with her? Or telling the truth? She felt numbness in her cheeks. It was the same numbness that overcame her many times in the past when she'd find herself plagued with social ineptness.

"So uh..." He brought the microphone pot down with his thumb and forefinger and raised another pot up that brought a hillbilly banjo duet to air. With his fingers on one hand lightly touching the surface of the pot, he pressed down on the keys of a nearby computer with this other hand. "What about you?" he asked. "What is this for you? An internship? You in school?"

"I go to Springfield U," Lori said, watching as he lowered the theme from "Deliverance" just in time for the first commercial spot to be played. She wondered how he could time everything so perfectly, and still be able to concentrate on talking to her. "One of my best friends..." she continued. "This girl Angela... She just got her first job doing reporting on radio for a local news network... and she's kind of an inspiration to me. I'm thinking about switching majors from science to communications."

"Science is the reason I'm here right now," he said, adjusting the gain pot.

"Why?"

"I was in the hospital for four months straight." He looked up at her. "Had a heart transplant." He studied her face for a response.

"Oh," she said. She nervously glanced away from him and tried to find something to focus her gaze on that would help her to take the news in better. Her eyes fell on his fingers. His nails were curved around his fingertips, which looked abnormally enlarged.

He noticed where her eyes had fallen. "What?" he asked.

"Um. Your fingers," she said. "They just look... Um..."

"Yeah." He let out a strained laugh. "It's part of my condition."

Her eyes fell to the floor. The words *faux pas* flashed in neon pink in front of her. She wished she could take both her show of ignorance and display of tactlessness back, but they were splattered like projectile vomit all over him.

"Still have marks on me," he said. He turned his body toward her, lifted his shirt to his chin, and traced his fingers along some pale tracks underneath his chest hair. He shook his head and let out a sigh. "I remember feeling so tired for so long. Used to get out of breath really easily. I'm feelin' so much better now."

"I'm glad."

"All 'cuz of science. Gave me a second chance here."

Up until then, Lori had been following in the footsteps of her older brother, a graduate student in the biochemistry department on the central Springfield campus. She had been mesmerized by all that he had been learning over the years, and she marveled at his unyielding energy and the long hours he'd dedicate to the laboratory. She fantasized that he was spending every minute of every hour, thinking and planning and plotting strategies that could lead to cutting-edge discoveries that could redefine life as it had up to then been known.

Seeing Nick, though, put her brother's hard work into a different perspective. She felt suddenly ashamed, realizing that she had never looked beyond the frivolous flash and glamour and self-fulfillment to see the true impact of that kind of work on a person's life. All of the future Bob Weir and Phil Lesh concerts Nick would still have the chance to go to, with his hair wrapped in a handkerchief and his tie dye shirt covered with beads, could be traced back to someone's late night toiling in a laboratory.

"You want to give it a try?" Nick asked.

"Give what a try?"

"This," he said, laughing. He pointed toward the mixing board.

"Oh." She hoisted herself onto his warmed, padded chair. With his guidance, she stiffly and awkwardly moved audio pots up and down and pushed buttons on verbal command. She could see the mechanics over time becoming rote, just as so many procedures she learned in biology lab had become with enough practice. Yet there was so much down time in between maneuvers, during which she was forced to listen to banter about Hedera Helix Selectas needing semi-shady locations and Peace Lilies requiring low lighting, that she was having trouble keeping focused on the clock.

"What happened to the break?" Nick asked. He had just returned from a vending machine on the floor below.

Lori looked over at the clock. Her hand hovered shakily over the microphone audio pot. "What should I do?"

Nick set an opened can of juice down, quickly leaned over her, and pressed down on a button. "Late break coming guys. Get ready." He waited a few seconds and with one hand slowly brought a bed of Ragtime music up under the hosts' voices. With the other hand, he pushed a lever that set the nearby computer loaded with commercials in motion.

"You're clear," he said to the invisible hosts before grabbing his juice can and guzzling it down.

"I'm sorry," Lori said. "I'm not too good at this, am I?"

"You're a little … slow."

Lori sighed softly.

"I'm just teasin'," Nick said, laughing.

Lori woke up early the following morning. She slipped on a loose pair of pajama bottoms, sat down on her dusty hardwood floor, and began to do a series of stomach crunches. She continued until the lactic acid build-up in her upper diaphragm reached unbearably painful levels. She swept her hand over the curvy surface of her bare stomach, hoping to detect a difference in its density, compared with how it felt ten minutes earlier. She stood up and walked over to her mirror, dropped her pajama bottoms to the floor, and stared in awe at the slightly flatter-looking silhouette of her torso. Could she have really lost unwanted fat in only fifteen minutes? Or was it just her posture creating an illusion?

Staring at the wild, untamed unibrow that sat like an awning over her eyes, she wondered what she would look like if she didn't have the means to occasionally keep all chaos in check, if she just "let herself go." She wondered whether if man had not created metal tweezers, pore-minimizing make-up, and electric shavers evolution would naturally select only fair-skinned, lean blonds for the purpose of non-alcohol-inspired procreation?

It was all a cruel joke, this sudden turn her body had taken just as she was finally starting to recover from the long-term repercussions of her adolescence, when her nose had shadowed her entire face and her fragile sense of self was particularly vulnerable to the verbal ice pick slayings typical of her unhinged Third Reich contemporaries. With wire-framed glasses and metallic braces added to the mix, she might as well have been strutting around naked in a cage filled with ravenous rabies-infected rottweilers with slabs of raw meat strapped to her ankles. She had emerged from junior high and had entered high school as traumatized and shredded as an unwanted, petrified fruitcake uneaten and re-gifted for decades. A fruitcake used occasionally as a mock football by young, restless children screwing around in basements on Hanukkah.

It was hard for Lori to envision herself as anything other than the fish-skinned, algae-infested, bog spawn creature from Hell her peers had convinced her she was and always would be. And not being able to see herself differently from how others had once seen her, she was left to wonder who in his right mind would want her? And how could she realistically be expected to want anyone in return who obviously wasn't in his right mind? She chose to believe what they led her to believe about herself, and she allowed their unmitigated attacks on the already deformed spine of her soul to contribute to her eventual emergence as somewhat of a broken spirit.

Rutherford was one of the few people Lori knew who could really relate to her. So could Angela. And it was heartwarming to her to know that they were both a part of her life and could share in the recollection of the misery of their respective pasts. But she hardly ever physically saw either one of them anymore, what with Angela's new reporting job keeping her busy at all hours of the day and night, and Rutherford's growing obsession with his laptop computer and preference to funnel any and everything that came to his mind into type-written, electronic messages.

From: SeriousSchmendrick4428@aol.com
Subject: he's back in black
To: LoriSolomon6697@yahoo.com
Dearest Lori,
I don't know if you remember or not, but when I was about 13 or 14, people would make my life miserable because I had braces and acne. I doubt if you know the

social horror and futility of weighing 320 (or was it 330?) pounds. I had a stretch of time where six straight girls said "uhh... no thanks" when I asked them out. SIX in a row! And these girls weren't exactly Victoria's Secret models, either. Uggg! I'm getting ILL just thinking about it!

I'm a "master of disguise," in case I never told you. The truth is I've never revealed my TRUE identity to anyone. Whenever you see me, I'm in my "big white dork" persona, but in actuality, I'm a shorter, skinny black guy.

Rutherford (a.k.a. The Tick)

Chapter 2

It is a long road that has no turning
Irish Proverb

Lori found Nick sitting quietly at the mixing board with an indecipherable expression on his face that could be interpreted as anything from mild boredom to fierce pensiveness. He briefly looked up at her. He quietly got up out of his seat and motioned for her to take his place.

"So you with anyone?" he asked a few moments after she sat down. Lori's hand was nervously perched over a microphone pot on the mixing board.

"Hmmm?"

"I asked if you were *with* anyone," he said, slowly. His midnight blue eyes locked with hers.

She looked down at the lever and was quiet for a moment. "Yes," she said, hesitantly.

"Yeah? What's his name?"

"Paul."

"Paul who?" he asked.

"Why do you want to know his last name? It's not like you'll know who he is."

"Just *tell* me," he said, a rough edge to his voice.

"Polansky."

"Paul? Paul Polansky? Hee, hee!" Nick moved his seat back a few inches and sat with his arms crossed over his chest, smirking at her.

"What's so funny?" she asked.

He grinned down at his folded arms and shook his head. "Nah, nothin'. I just feel like laughin'."

"Uh-huh," she said, thoughts of Paul filling her head and plaguing her with mind-numbing ambivalence. Over time, she had found herself in the transitory, undistinguished company of many Pauls. And her

15

insufferable frustration with them would inevitably cause her to flee from each one of them, their predictability, and their lack of complication. With her current Paul, she knew it was only a matter of time before she did the same. He wanted her, which meant only one thing: that he wasn't in his right mind.

"You look so cute right now, over there," Nick said. "Too bad you're spoken for."

Her face grew warm. She wasn't expecting the advance. Yet she felt anything but drawn to him. From the image of his long, kinky hair being set free from the worn rubber band that held it together, to the strange, grunge-like clothing he wore with all the mismatched, loud colors and stiff, uncomfortable-looking fabric, to the stray nose hairs peeking out from underneath his nostrils as he peered over her at the mixing board, she wondered if there was a girl on the planet that would actually find him attractive.

She felt badly for him.

"It's too bad we didn't meet sooner," he said. "If we did, we'd be screwing like bunnies."

Her shift ended late that Sunday evening. She swung the strap of her purse over her shoulder and started to walk out of the control room door.

"So do you wanna exchange e-mail addresses?" Nick cheerily asked her as she approached the threshold. "I got lots of jokes that I can send you."

"Uh, sure," she said, caught off-guard. She reached into her purse and ripped off a piece of a wrinkled envelope.

"Okay," he said. He pressed the scrap of paper against the wall behind him and scribbled away on it. "Now I better hear from you."

He had forwarded gags and riddles to her in rapid succession, as promised, and continued sending her scattered messages as the week wore on. Lori was intrigued by his sudden sustained attention, as well as pleasantly surprised that someone as strikingly *different* from her as Nick was actually reaching out to her. His look and demeanor reminded her of the boys in high school that she would always shy away from for fear that they would hit her with some spiteful, scathing remark as she passed by. These were the same boys that she would never see in her honors English or Social Studies classes, that she would never play chess or Backgammon with after school hours, and that she would never hear blowing into a tuba or French horn in the band wing. These were instead the boys that she would curiously stare down at from the bus window as it passed by the front stone wall of her high school, which was a notorious breeding ground for mind-altering hallucinogenics and drug dealers.

It was the following Sunday.

"So what happened to the jokes you were sending me?" Lori leaned over the mixing board and stared down at the word "audition" printed underneath a gain pot. Some of the ink was missing, making it instead read "auditio." She thought it made the word look foreign, like Spanish or Italian. "The e-mails just ... stopped."

"I dunno." Nick shrugged. "Haven't gotten any good ones lately to send, I guess." His voice was monotone and his eyes were averted toward an article in a trade magazine that he had lifted off of a shelf in the control room.

"Oh," Lori said. "Well ... I was enjoying reading them."

17

He continued perusing the magazine and said nothing. Lori slowly turned her body away from him and decided to try to shift her focus to the VU meters to make sure they were not pinning. She watched Nick curiously out of the corner of her eye, wondering what could be so interesting to him as to completely shut her out.

"What are you reading?" she asked, quietly.

He was silent.

"Nick?" She thought maybe he did not hear her. "Nick?" she said, loudly enough to give herself a jolt.

He remained motionless, merely flipping a page and continuing to read. "What?" he finally asked slowly, distractedly. He looked up at a small digital clock that sat above Lori's head and said, "Hey, are you ready for the break? It's coming up in a minute."

"Oh, yeah," Lori said, trying to force her attention away from him. "I think so." She pushed some buttons on a nearby computer and lined up a series of commercials for firing.

An hour or so of silence passed by, during which Nick continued to read, bewitched by the contents of his magazine. Almost unbearable stretches of boredom plagued Lori in between commercial breaks. She didn't understand why she found herself suddenly in the midst of a deep freeze with him, when he had otherwise been so warm and amicable just days earlier.

He slowly rolled his magazine into a mock telescope and started peering through it at her. "It's too bad you're taken," he said, lowering the magazine to his lap. He sat upright in his chair.

"And what if I wasn't taken?" she asked. She was grateful that at long last she was getting his undivided attention. "I'd just be one of many," she said teasingly. "I'd be lost in that endless line-up of girls you keep telling me you meet on Internet chat rooms."

"Yeah, but I'd put you right up there above 'em all," he said, smirking. "There's something about you, Lori."

Her curiosity about him was- to her surprise- beginning to grow. He was unusually confident for someone with his kind of rough and tumbled looks, subtly marred as they were by a small circle of shallow pockmarks on his right cheek and a slightly bulbous nose diminishing the size of his football-shaped eyes. Confident, and curiously untamable. What kind of spell, she wondered, was needed to make the cow chewing its cud stop simultaneously eyeing another patch of grass?

"We should do cyber sex sometime," he said, making a ring of keys dance around his forefinger. "E-mail me."

From: SeriousSchmendrick4428@aol.com
Subject: Horse fetish
To: LoriSolomon6697@yahoo.com

I'm in a weird, suspicious, introspective, and potentially psychotic mood. Hopefully I can turn this into something productive, but at this point I'm pessimistic.

I spent most of this afternoon reading the "Tao Te Ching" and searching for some sort of inner meaning, and I must admit that I'm making headway. But despite what I've read like "The sage does not act, therefore, he does not fail; he does not grasp, therefore he does not lose," I still feel like acting and grasping and basically punching someone in the face. I guess I'm just not cut out to be a "sage," but if I play my cards right I'm hoping that I can still get a government job eventually. Do ALL government positions require a drug test?

I've got two separate resumes done now. One is geared toward my Human Services experience, and the other highlights my B.A. in English and semi-extensive writing credentials (basically, my "writing credentials" are my nomination for the university poetry prize when I was in school). I picked up my resumes and a bunch of other job-hunting materials last Friday. So far, the only significant place I've sent my resumes is the upper shelf in my kitchen cabinet, so I don't accidentally spill beer and Jack Daniels all over them.

Rutherford

Lori had met Rutherford at Brimstone Park, a tiny stretch of softwood hemlock and pine trees and white cedar garden benches typical of the colonial southern New Hampshire village they both grew up in. They had started talking to one another on a day when Lori was hopping along a nearby tidal creek, Swallowtail gazing, and Rutherford was resting on a large granite stone reading gangster and serial killer collectible cards.

Occasionally, she would find a paperback book written about some occult-related topic that Rutherford would leave for her in her family's mailbox. He would set up camp with her in reputedly haunted burial grounds, and trudge with her through lonesome kettlehole bogs on the outskirts of town while reading the latest in his archeological digs of paranormal research and expert attempts at unraveling the mysteries of the supernatural. Rutherford seemed to be more impassioned over death than he was over the very life he was living, exhaustively examining the general futility of life at its mundane worst, and the liberation of death at its finite best. He spoke to Lori's bitter, ruthlessly reflective and increasingly pessimistic soul, and over time became the bitter, ruthlessly reflective and pessimistic mate her soul cried out for.

Despite the fact that Rutherford was only 22 years old, he predicted that he would eventually have to import a mail-order bride from overseas because he would never find an English-speaking woman who could tolerate him well enough to spend her life with him. In the meantime, he was considering providing his sperm to his friend Jill, a 25 year-old bisexual former exotic dancer and Wiccan who was contemplating conceiving a child out of wedlock that she planned on raising with her lesbian partner.

From: SeriousSchmendrick4428@aol.com
Subject: Creampuff
To: LoriSolomon6697@yahoo.com
Wherefore art thee? It seems that every time I change e-mail addresses nobody wants to write to me for weeks. So I'm back to my original address. May the Devil take me for a liar!
I'm giddy right now, because I think I have another hot date coming up with a local townie girlie this weekend. My friend Joe's new girlfriend hooked me up with this girl named Karla who just broke up with some guy like three months ago. She's, how shall we say, hot to trot. All night while we were hanging out, Joe kept nudging me in the side and winking, as if to say "you're in, you lucky bastard!" He and his girlfriend left around midnight, and I told Karla that she could "stick around" for a while if she wanted. By 12:02 I had her legs in the air, baby! I still can't believe how fast that happened. This chick, unfortunately though, is a piece of trash. She works at McDonalds. She's not in upper management, either. She's the one who hands you your Happy Meal at the drive-through. And she lives in a trailer.
Rutherford

Chapter 3

What you can not avoid, welcome
Chinese Proverb

Lori's internship at the radio station continued. She was assigned to start working some of her weekend shifts apart from Nick, and instead alongside a young woman named Helga. Like Lori, Helga had limited experience in radio and was training as she worked on the job. The conversations Lori had with her were short and focused only on the tasks at hand, which made for a very different atmosphere than the one Lori had grown accustomed to working alongside Nick. It also made for an atmosphere that she didn't enjoy nearly as much.

It was the evening after a long day of battling stream after stream of whiny complaints from Prima Donna talk show hosts, while taking care to press all the right buttons and shift levers in a timely fashion. Lori settled comfortably in her seat and looked over at Helga, ready to reflect on what she thought was a decent day's work, when the control room door opened. A frazzled, bearded black man stood a few feet away from the girls, pinching an inkless pen tightly between his thumb and forefinger. He tossed the pen angrily into a nearby garbage can.

"Now what was wrong with that transition?" Mitch asked, breathing fast and lifting a bag of popcorn to his mouth. His long, nimble fingers began shoving kernels between his lips as he stared angrily at them from behind his glasses.

"Too quick? Too slow?" mumbled Helga, brushing a long clump of blond hair away from her forehead.

"What? What did you say?" He was yelling now, and spitting pieces of popcorn.

Lori shifted uncomfortably in her chair. The unlabeled buttons and levers still looked confusing to her even though she had been in training now for quite some time.

"Too much music played before the liner?" Lori asked.

"No," he said calmly with a mouth full of fluffy kernels.

"Too quick of a switch from the last commercial to the bumper?"

He shook his head and said very slowly and loudly, "You did something that made the transition sound *bad*! Now what was it?"

"Something with the host's voice?" Lori asked.

He nodded his head and swallowed hard. "Now what about the host's voice? What did I train you to do with the host's voice?"

"You taught us not to overlap singing with the host's voice," Helga said, her eyes pointed down at the labels she was preparing for a stack of cassette tapes.

"You've got to be *in control* when you're at that goddamn board!" he yelled, continuing to spit popcorn out at them. "You *can't*, no matter *what*, get *distracted* when you're operating *the board*!!! If someone comes in and wants to talk to you, you say, 'Get the hell *out*!' You dig? If I come in and say, 'Hey, Helga, can I steal you away for a couple of seconds? There's something I need to go over with you...' You say, 'Mitch, *get the hell out*!' You've got to get the lion in your jaws, clench your teeth, and bite the living soul out of it, baby!" He smiled, nodded his head, and walked briskly out of the room, a trail of popcorn left behind him on the floor.

In a funny way, Lori felt herself drawn to Mitch. Just as he could be a growling bear with a stinging bite, complaining at times about the staff, or yelling curses at the mixing board when there was a loose connection causing dead air or the hotline had a short, he could also be soft and sweet like a kitten, remarking on Lori's "pretty brown eyes," and singing little jingles to her with an endearing grin on his face. It was similar to the kind of push-pull magnetism that Nick had; the kind that emanated from a constant enhancement and easing of tension.

It seemed as though just about every aspect of the station was beginning to take on a kind of aphrodisiac quality as time went on, like the drinking water had been tainted with Yohimbine or Spanish Fly. While Lori and Helga worked alongside one another at the mixing board each Saturday, their conversations gradually became more personalized and informal, their exchanges less polite and guarded. Helga began confiding in Lori about her lack of passion for her husband, her growing passion for a board operator named Burt, Burt's lack of passion for his wife, and his growing passion for her. And if Helga was not available at any point in time to divulge her secrets, then Lori could count on Burt to fill the void with his own personal accounts. Lori found herself caught in the midst of a developing affair, with pheromones flying wildly through the stale air of the control room and making her increasingly dizzy, detached, and confused.

From: NickWarren557@hotmail.com
oh baby…. maybe i could tease you in some hot talk…. i bet you'll like it a lot…. me and you talking dirty turning each other on…. yummy Lori…. the things we could do to each other…. oh baby…. i want you!!!!

Nick had started writing to her again, except instead of jokes, she found herself on the receiving end of Playboy Forum-like passages. While she didn't find herself interested in him the way that he seemed to be interested in her, she was still perversely interested in his interest. She was curious to know what he was going to say or do or write next to express it. The whole interplay seemed to her to be of a noninvasive nature, a kind of whirlwind of foolhardy erotica. She could just sit back, tease him with some mild flirtation of her own, and enjoy the newness and strangeness of it all.

From: Nick Warren557@hotmail.com
i wish i could kiss you all over from head to toe running my hands through your hair and slidin them up and down your body … feeling every hot inch of your tender flesh.… i bring my fingers to your … ohhh Lori ... to be continued …

She watched in fascination as his messages grew over time, in terms of perversion, bad taste, and unintelligibility. She looked at the propositions on her computer screen with a kind of jovial detachment. Yet she could still sense a cryptic danger lurking in the calm white spaces between his type-written, misspelled words. It was the kind of danger that Lori found hard to walk away from, even though she knew she should.

From: Nick Warren557@hotmail.com
well cutie ...☺
you miss my touch of my hands.… bet i cant wait to touch again!!!!!! you can too by the way.… i like touchin.… and yours are so sweet.… i wish i could see them now.… cant wait til we meet again
your admirer

It was another Sunday afternoon at the radio station. Nick sat passively in a chair by Lori's side, watching quietly as she tried unsuccessfully to connect the ISDN unit above her head.

"What is *wrong* with this thing?" she asked, pressing down hard on the buttons of a miniature keyboard. "Is this even *on*?" She stood up briefly and hovered over the equipment, trying to see if there was a loose wire or a plug out of a socket. "Springfield's going to need to connect with us for the top of the hour traffic report, and they won't be able to because I can't get the *stupid* ISDN to work! I mean, we've got a little time still. But I want to get it ready for them."

Nick continued to sit quietly, listening.

"This piss-ant operation's a completely half-assed set-up, you know that?" Lori ranted. "With all these ... ancient wires and cables ... that can literally get nudged by the tip of someone's sneaker under the mixing board and knock a 40,000-watt signal right off the air. The whole thing just doesn't make any sense. Every *day* it's something that's not working when it should!"

Nick slowly and silently raised himself up from where he sat. He moved closer to Lori and started to gently massage the knots of muscle in her neck and the small of her back. She was aware of all of the times that he had done this to her before, and that his hands had never wandered any further than a few generally neutral, sexless zones on her body. Yet this was different. Without any hint of a warning, he halted in the middle of his caresses to roughly sweep his hands over the front of her sweater and then jump away from her.

"What was that?" she asked. She was unable to contain the old familiar heat of embarrassment in her face.

"What?" he asked, soberly. "Hey, break's comin' in ten seconds. Get ready to pot down the mike and fire spots."

Lori looked at him for a moment, and then pushed a button on the computer to start airing commercials. After the last spot was played, a musical bumper smoothly transitioned the break into the next show segment. Nick leaned his face in toward her.

"I'm going to kiss you," he whispered. His hot breath tickled the side of Lori's jaw.

She slowly leaned away, feeling oddly removed from the reality of what he was proposing to do. Up until that moment, the idea of physically connecting with Nick was little more than a surreal concept harmlessly eyed at half an arm's distance as poorly written text on a computer screen.

"Come on," he said softly. He leaned more closely in toward her. "Come on," he whispered, while staring at her mouth, before pressing his lips passionately against hers. He continued kissing her until she pulled her body back and turned away from him.

He started to laugh. "I'm only teasin'," he said.

"Just teasing?" she asked. She shook her head. "You just kissed me."

He shrugged. With his hands placed uncaringly on his narrow hips, he pushed a few buttons quickly on the ISDN unit, bent over the mixing board, and pressed down on a lever.

"Traffic? You there?" Nick waited patiently for a response. "Traffic?"

"I'm here," answered a robust male voice over an intercom.

"We're connected and ready for you," Nick said. "Stand by."

Late that night, Lori sat staring out her living room window at the snow-covered streets and bushes. She noticed a veil of powder falling fast in front of a street lamp's glowing light. Paul was sitting opposite her on the couch, pressing buttons on a remote control with one hand, and rubbing the sole of her foot with the other.

That kiss ... She couldn't get her mind off of it. For the entire moment it lasted ... it had made her see and feel all of the things she had for so long dreamt of seeing and feeling. The intensity of two of the unlikeliest of souls coming together had engulfed her. It had seized her. It had held her. Time, for as long as the kiss had lasted, had stood still. And all of the evils that the passage of time was never able to erase had suddenly vanished like they had never even existed in the first place.

"Whatcha thinkin' about?" Paul asked, smiling at her intently.

"Nothing much," she lied. She continued to watch snowflakes drop from the sky and disappear into the frozen ground. Her mind was focused on only one thing: the kiss that was stolen earlier in the day in a seedy little control room at a Belchertown, Massachusetts radio station. The kiss that was forced on her by a young, punk, back street, oversexed, partying Dead Head that she hadn't even found herself remotely attracted to. It was the kiss that would whirl her into a state of suspended confusion and leave her staggering shamefully along the moonlit, stray cat-infested alleyway to unfathomable mayhem.

"I actually think I need some time to think about things," she said, feeling Paul's thumb come to a slow halt on the edge of her heel.

"You mean ... with us?" he asked.

She nodded.

"Is everything okay? Did I do anything?" he asked.

She shook her head and placed her hand gently on his arm.

In the time she and Paul had been together, Lori wondered if he even knew what she looked like from the neck down without clothes. Almost all erogenous zones had gone time and time again avoided and untouched, and the dropping of subtle hints would almost always lead to success that was only fleeting and forgotten by the time they next convened. As much as she loved being nurtured and cuddled and treated as a delicate, porcelain princess, there was this wild, ravenous part of her that seemed to want to be choked by a dog collar and led around on all fours like a dime store hooker.

"I know what I want," Paul said, lingering in her doorway at the end of their evening together. "My mind is made up. If you need more time, that's fine. But I want for us to be together."

She squeezed his hand, not knowing what else to do. Good-byes were always awkward, but angry good-byes were both awkward *and* painful. She didn't want there to be any pain. She didn't want there to be any anger. She just wanted there to be an ending. The same inevitable ending that she had suffered through so many times before.

"Sweet dreams," he said. He pulled away from her and disappeared into the darkness of her front lawn.

From: SeriousSchmendrick4428@aol.com
Subject: three balls
To: LoriSolomon6697@yahoo.com
I will probably NOT be seeing that girl from McDonalds again, hopefully. Unless I go to McDonalds, that is. I had fun with her last week, but that was a one-time thing. Period. I hate to sound like a stuck-up, pompous ass or anything like that, but that chick simply has NO CLASS. She looks presentable enough, but she's got this hoarse voice and a borderline hacking cough from smoking 3 or 4 packs of cigarettes an hour. Lori, I'm a dog. I admit it. I just wanted to get laid. Now, I want that

29

woman to DISAPPEAR! Anyway, I must go now. I'm a very busy man, and tonight I think I might finally break the 100,000-point level on Centipede.
Rutherford

Chapter 4

A spoon does not know the taste of soup, nor a learned fool the taste of wisdom
Welsh Proverb

From: Nick Warren557@hotmail.com
so i guess you really miss me now.... cant get enough of me out of your head.... hmmm ... i think i know what you need.... i know your ... must be screaming to be.... i would love to do that while i.... yah baby, you need it.... you want it.... im gonna give it to you....

It was another weekend. Nick lunged toward Lori. He chomped at her mouth, he placed his hands under her clothing, and he boldly turned his poorly-written cyberspace messages to her into a sinful, twisted reality that she had never before experienced.

"You're a good kisser," he said breathlessly. He mashed his lips forcefully against hers. The phone calls that poured in from listeners responding to the stale program being aired only perversely added to the intensity of the moment. He continued to press his lips hard against her mouth, his sweet breath caressing her cheek and jaw, his tongue wrestling with her own and sliding behind her front teeth. She softly bit his lower lip and slowly moved her mouth along the length of his bristly jaw and down toward his neck. She was just starting to feel the tangled hairs on his chest with the tips of her fingers as she moved her hands from the base of his neck toward his torso. His hands slid past her clavicle and swept over the neckline of her shirt, his fingers gently digging underneath the fabric. She soon felt the two of them melt into one as they wrapped

31

around each other in a tight embrace. She didn't want him to ever let her go.

"I'm gonna put you in my book some day," he said to her afterward, hovering over the pots of the mixing board and grinning devilishly at the VU meters.

Lori tried to imagine him disciplining himself enough to sit and pen a book, a book with proper grammar and spelling. She tried hard, but couldn't see it happening. Not him. Yet just the idea of him wanting to think and write about *her* forced a broad, endearing smile across her face.

From: Nick Warren557@hotmail.com
missin me yet.... i know your thinking of me.... you turn me on Lori
call me

She dialed his number.

"Hey." He answered immediately.

"I was asked to fill in for Burt at the radio station tomorrow night," she said. "It's a live remote, and I'm finishing up the last hour for him after my class."

"Yeah? Well, I'll be the one handling all the remote gear for the show. I might bring the equipment by the station tomorrow night," he said. "Maybe I'll see you there."

"Okay," she said, a hasty pang of anticipation shooting through her insides.

"Will ya make sure to wear a dress for me?" he asked.

The following evening, Lori nervously small-talked her way over a line feed through the last forty-five minutes of the live broadcast with one of the show's producers. Although she generally knew at this point how to operate the equipment by herself, she still liked the idea of having another human being physically present should the unforeseen and horrible happen. There was nothing that Lori feared more than the deafening sound of a long pocket of dead air, the feeling of not having the slightest idea of how to fill it, and the invariable and inevitable nasty verbal lashings that followed.

A few days earlier she listened to a first-time radio disc jockey on a major Springfield FM station play the same repellent pop song over and over again for five and a half hours in the absence of station identifications and commercials, all because he was left alone to try to operate faulty equipment. Some teenage listeners called in and made mock requests for the song so they could dedicate it to their friends, while others described how certain music caused them to have spontaneous orgasms and how listening to the station that evening had forced them to climax dozens of times within a span of several hours. All the disc jockey could do in between listening to the comments and waiting for an engineer to arrive was apologize profusely for the thousands of dollars he was costing the station in lost advertising revenue.

Lori's belly began to twist and turn and spasm shortly after she sat down in what had been dubbed the station's "hot seat," an appropriate label considering all that was bound to go awry once one sat down in it. She wasn't sure if the pain was caused by something that she had eaten that had not digested properly, or if it was the silent dread of what could transpire during her first independent shift at the station. All she knew was that she had to somehow will the discomfort away, to be able to make it through the next few hours before the station's signature sign-off. While the idle banter over the line feeds helped somewhat to calm her nerves, her churning stomach and wrenching intestines made time pass agonizingly slowly for her.

The broadcast was finally over, and she began airing a dusty stack of old previously recorded shows on cassette. She blew a gust of air from her mouth and pressed her fingers hard against the center of her bloated gut in a vain attempt to get the swelling and discomfort to move to a different part of her body. Looking outside the window of the control room, she could vaguely see a cold, wet mist forming in the glow of an oil lantern lighting the outside walkway. She glanced away from the light and toward the cloudy night sky, and her eyes fell on Nick Warren's parked lipstick red Ford Thunderbird against the horizon.

He assertively strolled through the door, sat down in a chair and said, "I heard your voice over the feeds and thought, 'hmmm, my *girlfriend's* there at the station.' Figured I'd pay a visit."

"I didn't think you'd actually come by tonight," Lori said. "I'm feeling kind of tired. Maybe you should just go home?" Her sickness, although uncomfortable, was making it easy to resist him. And this was refreshing in light of the fact that lately she had been feeling far too much like a chunk of modeling clay being kneaded and sculpted by his sweaty, busy hands. She didn't like the feeling of being out of control. And that was exactly what she realized she was, with Nick.

"No," he said, defiantly. "I want to stay here and admire your ..." He waved his hand expressively. "Your ... beauty."

"Please go home," she wheezed. *My beauty*, she thought. *Real sincere the way you put it.* She pulled an oversized sweater over her shoulders and crossed her arms. *Please go away. I'm not feeling well and even if I were... I... Please just go.*

"No," he said stubbornly. "Come over here." He reached out to her.

She hesitantly walked over to him.

He clutched the pockets of her jeans and slowly moved his hands up toward her waist and bosom. He gently pulled her body down toward him, and she straddled his hips with her legs and sat hard on his lap. She leaned her face in toward his and began softly kissing him on his lips and stubbly cheeks and neck.

Without a word, she succumbed.

From: Nick Warren557@hotmail.com
well i bet you been really thinkin of me

From: Nick Warren557@hotmail.com
call me here.... ill be waitin for your call hunny

A week had passed. It had been a week of justification, a week of rationalization, and a week of abstinence. Every day of that week, Lori dutifully sat in on her classes, automated, and emotionally detached. As she went through the motions, her thoughts revolved around the underlying impetus that placed her at Nick's mercy every weekend. She figured the driving force could best be summed up as a cry for freedom. Freedom that she knew could lead to either mind-numbing cycles of constant yearning and agonizing disillusionment, or delicious enlightenment.

Instability and restlessness were not going to disappear so long as the fear of stepping upon the unsteady platform of risk paralyzed her. She had already taken the first step in breaking free from the confines of the mundane, once she realized that she needed to get out there. Wherever "there" was, that was where she felt she needed to be. Even if it was just to get a taste of "there" while still staying within the safety zone of "here," Lori felt that it was critical that she do so, if for no other reason than to feel like she was alive.

That weekend, she and Nick slithered like slimy snakes on the soiled and worn rug of the station's fusty basement. Her hands moved fast and furiously across his hairy back and up and down the sides of his solid, narrow torso. She tried pulling his body, tight and muscular, closer, so that she could hug him, and somehow ... some way ... get all the aching, wrenching passion she was feeling to diffuse out of her own body and into his. The light-headedness she felt, like she could easily faint from complete and utter loss of control, was overwhelming her. How could she feel so much for someone? And how could she feel so much for someone that she felt like she barely even knew?

She skulked through the darkened corridors of the old building afterward, feeling odd and confused, and at the same time peculiarly jubilant. Nick had tapped into something inside of her, a very primal part of her sexuality that others in the past may have come close to but never hit the central core of. She felt energies that had been pent up her whole life come rushing forth, carrying with them unleashed fantasies and leaving behind an ironic sense of peace and fulfillment.

Yet that night at the station would be just one of many fiery hot nights lying ahead of her, with an icy cold chill in the air willing any feelings of composure and serenity away. The nights would come and go fleetingly, so fleetingly that at times she was actually left feeling *dumbfounded*, wondering why she had allowed this gremlin of the night to feast on her flesh according to unspoken terms that only he understood and abided by.

Nick would learn whether or not Lori was working closing shifts on Sunday evenings at the station. He would visit, and slip his arms possessively around her shoulders, and then turn otherwise unremarkable evenings … unchaste. He would then leave like an endorphin-high actor taking a quick bow after a lengthy performance and leaping off the stage.

But there was an unsettling side of him that was apparent to her even long before his "visitations" became increasingly businesslike as though he were some kind of hired gigolo. It was a part of him that ironically seemed to lure her into his baneful clutches even deeper.   Just as quickly as he would lather her with soul-penetrating attention, his eyes would avert and his posture would change and his entire aura would turn frosty and gray.   It was as though he were a catatonic schizophrenic slipping into and out of a trance. And even more disturbingly, Lori found that, over time, she was becoming drawn just as much to the hollow echoing darkness as to the occasional bright warming light.

Something was terribly wrong.

From: SeriousSchmendrick4428@aol.com
Subject: the Di is cast
To: LoriSolomon6697@yahoo.com
My honest gut (big beer gut) instinct tells me that if you think there's a problem, you'd better nip it in the bud (or is it "butt"? I could never figure that one out and I've been too embarrassed to ask someone) right now.
Rutherford

Time passed.   Lori and Nick were no longer scheduled to work together on weekends, and so they did not see each other for weeks. While a part of her longed to see him, another part of her was relieved not to. There were too many questions running through her head and not nearly enough answers. Where was it all to go? How long would it continue? How would she feel about it in time? How did she feel about it *now*?

Wouldn't the simplest move on her part be to settle in with Paul Polansky, a firm and beefy box-spring mattress positioned underneath her for strength, support and leverage? Once in place, couldn't she blanket herself with whatever adventure or excitement she desired, *without* the danger?

There was a pacifying and sleepy comfort in knowing that Paul could be there for her, with open arms for her to embrace, and his quiet, unthreatening nature, and his nice, pleasant ways. Yet if Lori were to be completely honest she knew that deep down inside her, Paul's Hallmark card style tenderness could only chip away so much at the thick scab that had for a long time encased her scalloped heart. She seemed to find herself, time and time again, grasping for the unfamiliar, lunging toward uncertainty, tirelessly sifting through desert sand in search of an oasis. It was like trying to calm a restlessness, to fill a dark emptiness. Yet why was it that what she seemed to always reach out for ended up being more barren than what she was trying to fill?

Chapter 5

Friends are like fiddle strings, they must not be screwed too tight
English Proverb

From: SeriousSchmendrick4428@aol.com
Subject: 3.1415 ... infinity ...
To: LoriSolomon6697@yahoo.com
"Asu49991 could take its place alongside others in a new class of small molecular compounds that selectively destroy cells with abnormalities." --Robert Solomon, Ph.D.
That's some funny stuff. Sounds like your brother's had a breakthough. Hey, does he know that you have a friend named Rutherford who hasn't showered in almost 11 days?
I'll speak with thou later.
Rutherford

Lori decided to pay her first visit in a long time to Angela, who was residing in the cramped attic of her parents' 1925 Colonial along with her four de-clawed and neutered cats. She was led up a long flight of wooden stairs that guarded a corner of an unheated garage, and that led to a small A-frame room with nothing but Angela's four-post bed and a dresser propped up against a window. A lengthy, narrow crawl space, filled with rumpled clothing and linen, led from the attic into the bedroom Angela's sister had grown up in. Her parents were just a yodel away in their master bedroom down the hall.

Lori had met Angela the year before at school during a college theater production of *The Pirates of Penzance*, in which they both had been allotted minor parts. In the backstage dressing room one evening, several hours before their first rehearsal, Lori had found the raven-haired, buxom Angela sobbing loudly into the silky scarlet sleeve of a costume hanging on a nearby rack. While trying to console her, Lori learned that Angela was devastated over not having landed the role of Mabel, and that she had always been the star of every play she had ever acted in since the age of six and a half. And how *dare* this particular troupe overlook her vast experience in theatre and hard-earned credentials- which arced back to her *elementary* school days for heaven's sake- in favor of someone Angela *knew* was far inferior in terms of vocal projection, demeanor, and overall onstage presence?

Perhaps it was her brazen sassiness that made Lori feel instantaneously spiritually and intellectually connected. Perhaps it was the things Angela said and the amazingly open way that she said them that spoke directly to Lori, and that made Lori want to know more of her. Lori didn't know why, exactly, but she felt an instant kinship.

"So Lori," Angela said, shutting the door to her closet-sized bathroom to keep the cats from wandering in. "You'll never guess what station I've been assigned to."

"Belchertown."

"Springfield Regional Broadcasting Network just took on five new local clients, Belchertown being one of them. They've got me doing their midday news." She walked over to her bed and sat on its edge. "Take a seat," she said to Lori, pointing to a rattan chair perched against a wall. "Guess who's taking my feeds?"

Lori's heart started to pound.

"That guy Nick, would you believe it? You're right about him being a flirt."

"What do you mean?" Lori asked.

"He's just… so flirty… asking me what I look like, inviting me out to Belchertown… He sounds kinda cute. What does he look like?"

"No one you'd be interested in," Lori said, feeling the muscles in her neck tense up. She tilted her head from one side to the other and tried to massage the tightness in her shoulders away.

"Did you know that he had a heart transplant? I can't imagine… Did he ever tell you about that? I mean, that's some pretty heavy stuff. It's hard to picture, someone his age, going through that."

Lori stopped kneading her neck muscles and let her hands flop down into in her lap. She cusped them, and started to make her thumb nails wrestle with each other.

"He said doctors are giving him *ten years*, plus or minus a few," Angela said, her voice shrill. "Could you imagine?"

Lori shook her head quietly.

"What's wrong, Lori? You got quiet on me."

Lori's eyes dropped to the floor.

"It is something that has to do with Nick? Lori…" Angela said. "Did you *do* anything with that guy?"

"Yeah," Lori said, continuing to stare down at her feet. "But it's over. I mean, since we stopped working together on weekends, I haven't seen him. And I haven't heard from him. And I really don't care. Or honestly feel like talking about it. If you don't mind."

"Well, Lori…" Angela stood up and walked over to her dresser. She picked up a pilled teddy bear and began playing with its paws. "It's not like I'm really all that *interested* or anything like that. It was just flirting. *Light* flirting. And it's not like it'd ever *go* anywhere. Not with someone like him." She placed the bear back on the surface of the dresser and turned to face Lori. "Hey, come with me. I want to show you something."

Lori followed Angela through the crawl space leading into her sister's old bedroom. They tip-toed past the master bedroom where Angela's mother was sleeping and they headed into Angela's parents' living room where a big beautiful parlor grand piano sat to one side of a soapstone fireplace.

"Listen to this, Lori," Angela said. "You listening?"

"Ready."

Angela played Lori a sweet-sounding tune she had written several days earlier. Her singing, only slightly off-key, was still beautiful to Lori's ears.

"I have to tell you," Angela said. "I feel completely foolish for having sung to you just now. I must have sounded like complete crap. I've got this morning frog in my throat, plus I've got a little cold ... I'm feeling so self-conscious ... like you're just being polite saying you liked it ... Could you even tell that I *can*, in fact, sing? I sang the song for my dad last night, and it sounded infinitely better ..."

"It was one hell of a lot better than anything I could ever do," Lori said.

"Yeah, but you see, that sounds ... like you don't really think it was that good. Otherwise, you'd be more enthusiastic. I mean, if it's 'a hell of a lot better than you could ever do,' that might not be saying much because according to you, you can't sing or write music at all. See what I mean? So now I feel even worse."

"Angela, I can sing a *little*. I mean, I haven't had any professional training, but I don't think I completely suck at it."

"So what you're saying ... and I *promise* to drop it after this ... is despite my 'morning throat' you can at least tell that I have a decent voice and can carry a tune?"

"Yes!"

"Look, I'm sorry to be so needy. I have *no* confidence in *anything* right now. The last time I got together with my coworker Myrna from the news hub and were talking about looks, she said she couldn't really remember what her first impression was of mine. She said she figured she thought I was attractive, but that the more she got to know me, the more attractive I became to her. So ... what did I do with that? Interpreted it as she probably thought I was really plain-looking or even ugly *until* she got to know me, and my personality shone through! I obsessed about it for *days*... and it's still on my mind. I'm telling you, all anyone has to do these days is look at me cross-eyed and I *freak out*! I e-mailed a *priest* today asking for some kind of spiritual guidance. You have no idea how on the edge I feel."

Lori nodded quietly.

"I honestly think that you're more secure than I am, Lori. I mean, I think we're a lot alike, but I go off the deep end, and you don't. I'd love to know how you keep yourself 'sane.'"

Lori smiled, and pressed down on some black and white keys on the far left-hand side of the piano. "Sane?" Lori echoed. "That's a strong word to use for someone like me."

"Well, compared to *me* you're sane!"

Lori laughed. "Maybe I'm just... I don't know. I mean, Angela, I also get accused of thinking and worrying too much about things. Caring too much about things. Like what people think of me. What I think of them. Wanting everything and everyone around me to be okay all the time."

Angela nodded.

"But ... as much as I feel this like ... need to always try to make sense of things, and dissect each and every thing that's going on that's not sitting right with me… and then try to *make* everything right… every so often I need to get outside of my head for fear of being completely taken over by it."

"Uh-huh."

"I try throwing myself into things. Just about anything I can think of that'll get my mind off of whatever it is I'm likely to be obsessing over."

"I *try* to do that! I honestly *do*, Lori! All right- for example, I *love* to read, so when I find myself getting worked up, I try throwing myself into a book. But then I find myself drifting away, to the point where I end up reading the same page a hundred times! It's *so* frustrating, Lori. You don't know how much it *sucks* to be me. I don't *want* to be like this, but it feels like I can't help it."

"You know, I see people out there not giving a flying you-know-what about anything, and I think about how happy those people seem to be, and how miserable people like you and I *know* we are, and I think… something just isn't right here," Lori said. "Maybe the trick to enjoying life is just not taking it as seriously as we both have a tendency to?"

"I think we just need to lighten the f- up."

Chapter 6

*There is no disguise which can hide love for long where
it exists, or simulate it where it does not*
Francois de La Rochefoucauld (1613-1680)

From: SeriousSchmendrick4428@aol.com
Subject: mac and chizeese
To: LoriSolomon6697@yahoo.com

I am just beginning to realize that all I do is work, get
buzzed often, and watch a worthless world fly by me. All
I ever come home to are a computer screen, a plate of
cheese, and a bottle of beer. I conduct my love/sex life
more like a series of isolated commando missions than
anything normal or healthy. I see a target, I STRIKE,
and I go back into hiding. I have NEVER been involved
with a girl that I actually gave a damn about, although
I've tried to convince myself otherwise. It's always about
ME. I'm starting to wonder if I'm even CAPABLE of
giving a damn about anyone. This, of course, has major
advantages, like the fact that I've got a bulletproof
emotional construct. Unfortunately, it also means that I
am depriving myself of feeling anything "beautiful" in the
interest of self-preservation. I'm afraid that I'll meet
someone I actually like, and when she ultimately finds
out what an irresponsible, immature, and self-centered
BASTARD I am, she'll tell me to take a hike, and wise
she would be to do so. I can't even figure out who I am.
I've got this big ego, and yet I'm consumed with self-
loathing. I think everyone else is so screwed up, and yet
I'M the one who probably needs therapy. I used to think
I was detached from the world, but in fact, I am
detached from myself.

I'd like to meet Angela at some point. Tell me more
about her. Can she appreciate the beauty and stench of
a perfectly aged Alsacian Munster cheese? Does she

smoke weed? What have you told her about me? Hmmmm... Did you tell her that I'm a self-taught culinary genius and a badass on Pac Man? I'm no slouch with Donkey Kong, either. Believe me. I know girls are turned on by guys my age who do nothing but cook and drink beer and play video games, right? WHOA!
Rutherford Gimby

Lori had never been one to indulge in self-help books, spiritual enlightenment seminars, vibrational metal tong and puck soul healing workshops, Disciples of Jesus Jew bashing gatherings, Tantric sex orgies, group hugs, or anything else that the few or the many seemed to be drawn to as attempts to pull meaning into their lives and achieve inner peace. Angela had apparently nibbled at some of these options from time to time, much in the same way as a rat samples a crumb before engulfing the entire morsel of food for fear it is a toxin that it would be unable to regurgitate. She made sure to regularly give Lori the synopses of any interesting and relevant *Cosmopolitan* magazine articles she'd come across, like those on repeatedly attracting and becoming attracted to retards, or the latest of her self-help purchases: a forty dollar, hard-covered, Ph.D.-scribbled, "Women Who Love Women Who Love Men Who Have Mothers Who Did Not Love Them and Who Screw Over the Women Other Women Love but Shouldn't as These Women are Screwed and Hopeless." And she was also good about letting Lori in on the priveleged details of her most recent, and most disappointing, ten dollar, health insurance-covered session with some "impartial" stranger with a personal code of ethics that Angela believed could easily spill over and turn a supposedly objective view point into one potentially damaging, sorry ass line of brain tenderizing garbage.

Lori, herself, just couldn't bring herself to lean on any one crutch on any regular basis and believe that this was what would exorcise the seemingly unyielding angst that came with believing one was hopeless and fated to a lifetime of complete, irreparable mayhem. Her feeling was that once any good vibes from shared anecdotes inevitably dissipated, she would still be left with her own very unique demon-spawn foibles that only shared a skin-deep resemblance to the foibles of others.

And yet, she still found herself in times of woe drawn to her friends like metal to a magnet, and she salivated like Pavlov's dog every time they opened up their lives to her and dished out the same level of intimacy that she would freely and gladly dish out to them. It was true that in essence they were all most likely co-enablers of each other's mayhem serving only to mask their pain in a misery loves company kind of way. And perhaps by masking the pain they were actually inadvertently perpetuating it. But they continued to look very much forward to exchanging their stories and digging their philosophical heels deep into the quicksand of their dysfunction. After all, it was far cheaper than therapy, and a hell of a lot more fun.

From: SeriousSchmendrick4428@aol.com
Subject: golden shower with self-proclaimed moral fiber
To: LoriSolomon6697@yahoo.com
I'm drunk. It's almost four in the morning. I got your e-mail about calling here, but my roommate is a complete MORON about not giving me my messages. He never mentioned a WORD about it. He just erased it from the machine. That's unbelievable. Anyway, one reason

I've been playing the "absentee" role lately is because I've placed some ads in various "personals" sections online, looking for girls to talk to, and I've gotten so many responses that I am positively OVERWHELMED. The screwed-up thing, so far, is that the ONLY girl that I've been "chatting" with, and that I'm the most interested in and intrigued by, lives in Kansas City, which is not a geographic advantage for making any kind of "love connection." We've just been talking about life and all that. She's a very interesting and intelligent girl, and we've got so much in common that it's downright frightening. I'd better just drop it, now, lest I start to sound like the shortsighted, ignorant clown that I am.

I will speak with you shortly, of course, and I may need your womanly advice about how to handle some things. I actually saw my ex tonight, very briefly, and I thought about asking HER for some advice, but screw that. She's got a new boyfriend, who I'm told is a complete dick. Unbelievable. You see, Lori, THAT'S the problem. No matter HOW much you try and deny it, the fact is that MOST girls are NOT interested in guys like me. I'm not saying ALL girls. I'm just saying "most" girls. I've never met any of your boyfriends, Lori, but just let it be known that, not to stroke your ego, I've always felt that you were way too smart and perceptive to fall into that "jerk-lover" syndrome, so I'm not saying that YOU like jerks, but MOST girls do, and don't even think about denying it … If I'd have treated my ex like a piece of trash, I'd be in bed with her right NOW, and that's a FACT, so put that in your pipe and smoke it. I'm just kidding about the pipe, but NOT about the way that girls are largely attracted to DICKS. I don't care what anybody says … Nice guys always DO finish last, and you can take THAT to the bank. It never ceases to amaze me when I think about how many stupid, arrogant, self-absorbed asses I've known in my life that had girls falling all over them... some girls I actually respected. Can you tell what a frustrated, lonely, angry bastard I am becoming yet?

Anyway, I'm tired, I have a headache, and my feet are beginning to stench. I haven't washed these socks in a week. Showering seems futile and tedious and ultimately conformist. Lord, I'm pathetic...

I've got to go, but we'll talk expediently. Just don't bother leaving me any messages, because there's only a 50/50 chance that I'll get it, anyway.

Yours,

Rutherford (a.k.a. Johnson Longwood)

Lori flocked to Rutherford's apartment in Portsmouth to seek solace amongst his proudly displayed pile of belly button lint in the corner of his shower, petrified clumps of black bearded growth lining his entire bathroom sink basin, and ten week-old fungus- and mold-covered coffee cake in the center of his kitchen table. He loosely tied the back of his cooking apron while she talked, and hunched over a kitchen counter covered with recipe books and an array of pots, pans, spices and vegetables. He began to lightly dust an ensemble of chicken strips with pan searing flour, making sure to nod every so often to let Lori know that he was paying attention to her. With a spray of olive oil weakly smoking in a pan behind her head, she talked to him about meaning, and how it seemed as though some people didn't seem to have a need for it when it came to relationships. Where was the meaning, she asked, in a union that was strictly of the physical nature, propelled mostly by ego, sustained primarily by hormones? A union that was more analogous to a killing by camouflaged hunters in deer-infested woods; a union that could very well end up torn apart, its vulnerability jutting out as a prized capture on a whitewashed wall?

"Lori," Rutherford said. "The pathologies involved here aren't important. And my theories are so twisted that even I don't understand them."

Lori looked quizzically at him. *What?*

"The important thing," he continued, carefully setting the chicken slices on the pan to cook, "is that you obviously get rather turned-on by guys who aren't afraid to shower you with sexual commentary and bold-faced aggressive behaviors, right? Correct me if I'm wrong about that."

She remained quiet.

"Look," he said. "It all boils down to 'I want to get screwed like a dog, and Paul isn't doing that.' Right? Of course I'm right! As for an insight into the 'male mind,' you'd better sit still, as what I'm going to say may offend you. Nick Warren has no concern for you whatsoever. He doesn't *care*! He, I *guarantee* you, is lying around his home and thinking about how easy and bizarre it was to get between your legs by simply flashing his weenie at you. That's the way guys think, Lori. You showed him vulnerability, and he simply capitalized on it."

Lori shifted uncomfortably in her chair, her elbow brushing a piece of petrified, once-buttered toast lying on a nearby plate. "I think there's more to it than that," Lori said. She forcefully pushed the plate away from her end of the table.

"No there isn't!" Rutherford looked at her incredulously. "Trust me, Lori, you're completely wasting your time and emotions worrying about 'closure' from any guy that you've ever taken as a partner only for the purpose of sexual liberation," he said. "They don't *care* who you are. It might sound simplistic, but I'd gladly debate any mother like Nick on the matter." He removed the pan of caramelized chicken from the stovetop and sprinkled some parsnips around it before placing it inside the heated oven below. "He might rant and rave about this crap and try to save his face in mixed company, but once any ladies were out of the room, he'd giggle and nudge me in the ribs and say 'Yeah! It was so *easy*! You know!' I'll bet every cent that I have in the bank that that's what would happen. Now, I've only got like *six* dollars in the bank, but that doesn't diminish my conviction."

Lori sat quietly, watching Rutherford obsess over the lumpy consistency of a tub of chicken gravy. He carelessly bustled about his kitchen as though there was no one there but him and his organic food and seasonings and cookbooks, and Lori continued to watch him without saying a word.

"The only advice I have for you," he continued, "is to learn how to get Paul to pull out the dog collar and give you a good animalistic *screw*. Right? Tell him that you don't care about the cuddly-wuddly crap. There's nothing *wrong* with that!" He removed the chicken from the oven and placed it back on the stove next to a bottle of basting oil. "As for Babette, I've thought *a lot* about what *she* is up to when I'm not around. I'm not stupid, and I'm not naïve. With Babette, I don't trust her, but the irony of my mistrust is that I *do* trust that she'd tell me about it immediately if she was with someone else. And the ultimate irony is that *I don't care!*"

Lori was home again, mindlessly thumbing the pages of an assigned chapter in her sixth edition microbiology textbook. She wished its contents were more personalized, more of the type of subject matter she could relate to. She didn't want to think about bacterial flagella and prokaryotic versus eukaryotic cells. She wanted to think about life, and death, and love, and lust, and pain, and angst, and emotion. Maybe she'd switch her major to psychology.

Her phone rang.

"Hey."

"Who's this?" she asked.

"Nick."

It had been weeks.

"Oh, hey," she said, her fingertips numb against the receiver. "What do you want?"

"So uh … I was … wondering what you uh … meant by a certain … *joke* you wrote on one of the logs at the station."

"What joke?" she asked. Her heart was rapping violently inside of her chest, shaking her ribcage. The last thing she had remembered drawing on a radio log was a series of arrows with teasing phrases like "turn the page for a surprise," and "keep going," and "you're getting warmer." On the last page that was preceded by another arrow and another tease was the word "SUCKER!"

"You know," Nick said, his voice getting softer. "No more Dick on Sundays," he whispered.

"I wrote that a long time ago." She found herself suddenly having difficulty catching her breath. "Just white it out."

"So what did you mean by that?" he asked.

"Well…" She swept a sweaty hand through her hair and tossed her textbook onto a bare couch cushion. "I was producing Dick Soho's call-in dating show on Sundays, it got cancelled because there were no callers, and I felt badly about it."

Silence. After stumbling and fumbling for what to say next, he finally said, "I just figured I'd call to harass you."

"Thanks," she said. "Look, I have to go."

"Okay."

"Bye."
"Bye."

From: SeriousSchmendrick4428@aol.com
Subject: Guess who's coming to dinner
To: LoriSolomon6697@yahoo.com
Dearest,
Nick has no regard for you. I guarantee you that you have not heard the last from him, nor will you ever hear the last from him, as long as you entertain his overtures in ANY way whatsoever. When you heard his voice on the phone, you should have hung-up immediately. However, you didn't do that. Don't you see how predictable this is? Jesus, woman, wake the hell up! I'll tell you right now, point blank, what I think of this. I think that this guy has absorbed such information about YOU and your interpretations of sex and relationships to fulfill his own lecherous end. Lori … Wake up. Nick sees you as a horny little honey that he can keep on the side to manipulate for his own personal pleasure. This crap is as easy as two-plus-two. Wake up, god dammit, you can't possibly be as foolish and gullible as you're sounding. You can rant and rave all you want about wanting to be done with those encounters with Nick, but the fact is that you are still excited about it all, and on some weird level you want them to continue. Tell me I'm wrong. Go ahead … TELL me I'm wrong.
NOT!
Rutherford

Lori was called in on a weekday to voice a commercial for the radio station. This was a rarity, as the station mostly used male voices for spots, and there weren't many spots to voice to begin with.

Over time, more and more of the original radio staff were being recruited to fill full-time positions for a new business-oriented format that was being launched at the station. Lori sat on a paisley chenille sofa near a maze of newly erected office cubicles in the station, silently marveling at how much more structured, sterile and corporate the building was beginning to look. The office outside the closed production studio door was vacant, apart from Nick sitting quietly at his desk with his back to her. She noticed that he had lobbed off his frizzy ponytail, an obvious attempt to try and blend in better with the highfalutin, impervious social infrastructure of the place, run as it was now by cosmopolitan, suit and tie, Wall Street Journal types. It was the most revolutionary of takeovers by the carbon copy Boston Blue Bloods, with their cappuccino-stained ceramic mugs artfully decorating the edges of their cubicle wall-divided desktops, and their scores of circling, flirtatious, waif-like administrative staff. It was a black and white contrast to Metro West Hepcats like Helga and Burt, who drank from striped paper cups and whose creative, libidinous energies could never be confined to the boundaries of an office cubicle.

Nick said nothing to Lori as she quietly continued to sit on a thick cushion of the couch, waiting to be called into the production room. He merely maintained a Pompeii frozen posture while staring intently at the screen of his computer and typing. He acted as though she were not even present in the room. But Lori knew that Nick was very much aware of her, perhaps more aware than he had wanted to be.

The game was on. Lori cleared her throat. "Do you want to hear a joke I heard?"

Nick's head turned, and a toothy smile grew on his face. "You wanna see it?"

"No," she said, with a laugh. "I asked you if you wanted to hear a *joke*. What would make you think I was referring to 'it'?"

54

"Well it's here anytime you want it," he mumbled casually, returning to his typing.

The production manager's face appeared in the doorway of the studio, and he motioned for Lori to come inside. She sashayed past Nick's desk, where he had resumed his veneer of engrossment and importance. She slowed her pace some, but did not look at him. Not directly. He was kept only in her peripheral vision, just as he seemed to be lingering only in the frayed fringes of her life.

She promptly finished her session and emerged from the recording studio. Rounding a corner, she longingly eyed Nick's empty chair and vacated workstation. She drew a deep breath, slowly let the air out of her lungs, and gently swept her fingertips across the surface of his desk as she made her way out of the building.

Back at home, Lori lay in her bed, just starting to drift off to sleep. She lifted a Greek philosophy book fanned out on her chest and set it down on some floorspace near her bedside. She turned her body to one side, tucked her legs up in a fetal position, and thrust her arms underneath her pillow. Her breathing deepened and the hum of a digital clock on her nightstand grew fainter and fainter.

Her phone was ringing. She was jolted awake.

"Hello, Lori? It's Nick." It was like a creature from a monster movie suddenly coming to life again after looking as though it had been killed sufficiently for the closing credits to begin rolling.

"Hi," Lori said, her lungs airless from her throat suddenly closing in on itself.

"I just called to see how you were doing."

"Aw … Really?"

“And I was wondering if you wanted to drop by the station sometime and keep me company.”

Chapter 7

He that seeks trouble never misses
English Proverb

From: SeriousSchmendrick4428@aol.com
Subject: Help this ...
To: LoriSolomon6697@yahoo.com
Lori, I have a weird complex that I'm trying to figure out. I was discussing it with my friend Joe last night, so I might as well discuss it with you.

You see, there are certain situations in which I have a tremendous amount of confidence, almost to the point of being arrogant (well, I guess it IS to the point of being arrogant, actually). When I'm in that "zone," there is nothing I'm afraid to do, say, or try. I have absolutely no fear, and absolutely no regard for potentially negative consequences. This is the attitude I have around certain girls (like Babette, and a few others that I probably never mentioned). However, there are times when I'm basically a pussy. I feel ugly, stupid, and worthless. I often feel that way when I'm surrounded by strangers, which is why I almost NEVER go out anywhere in public, or when I'm in unfamiliar situations. Every so often, it's like my mind starts focusing on every single little imperfection about myself that I can think of ... I've got a bad haircut. I don't dress well. I wear glasses. My teeth aren't perfect. My voice is goofy. I'm overweight, etc. etc. etc. I can hardly think of a word to say. It's like I regress to the point of being an insecure teenager who can't get a date for the school dance.

Where am I going with this? I don't even know, but that's the deal. It's like I'm drawn to, and I excel in, negative situations, but when something potentially GOOD might happen I completely convince myself that it's hopeless and I'd better run the other way.

So what do I do? Go into therapy? On the other side of the coin, why are some girls so drawn to me even though I'm an emotional train wreck? It's a paradox, I tell you.

Do you think I'll ever be able to meet your friend Angela?

Anyway, I will speak with thou in a fortnight, for I have been pitched in battle and am weary for a mug of ale and a wench to relieve my weary burden...

Rutherford

From: AngelontheAirwaves3254@hotmail.com
Subject: Re:
To: LoriSolomon6697@yahoo.com

LL/SF,

I had a date last night, and it sucked. The guy was just so, I don't even know how to describe him. Just ICKY is the only word that comes to mind.

I'm feeling so lonely and vulnerable right now. It seems like most of the guys I'm attracted to just DO NOT look back at me. For whatever reasons, they don't. When I was on the thin side, guys said I was too skinny. Now that I'm on the heavy side, they say I'm too heavy. And even when I was "just right" in most peoples' eyes, guys just never really responded to me, sexually. Take my good friend, Carl- the one who chose Stephanie (the Bitch) over me. He always told me he looked at me more as a sister than anything else. My friend Robbie always said the same thing. Yet, I would have gone out with either of these two guys in a heartbeat. I don't know what it is I lack- but I have never, ever been the type who could "have any guy I wanted." Not even close. That is why I've always felt like I had to take whatever was available. Over the years, when I'd go out to clubs and bars with friends, I would inevitably end up feeling invisible- like the ugly stepsister. I don't put myself in situations like that anymore ... But it left an indelible mark on me. One time I was really interested in this guy named Pete. My friend Karen tried to fix us up ... But you know what he said? "I really like Angela, and she's not bad-looking, but I want someone REALLY attractive." To this day, I can't believe Karen TOLD me this, but I pushed her for a reason, and she finally caved in. Later in my life, another guy said virtually the same thing. That he wanted someone beautiful, not just cute.

So, in sum, I've gone through life feeling like I really did not have a choice. I'd let them choose me ... and be grateful that every now and then, I was chosen.

By the way, is your friend Rutherford still interested in meeting me?

Angela

Rutherford and Lori shared a cold pale lager before meeting Angela at a nearby Springfield pub. Angela stood near a crowded bar, clutching a glass of sparkling Merlot and smiling broadly. She threw her free arm around Lori.

"Lesbian lover!" Lori exclaimed, hugging her back.

"Shhh!" Angela giggled. "People know me here." She swept past Lori and enthusiastically shook Rutherford's hand. Angela had recently begun doing live, nightly newscasts at a local cable station several notches above public-access, and because of her newfound local celebrity had become considerably image conscious.

That day, Rutherford had looked a little different to Lori, with pink color in his cheeks from long mushroom-hunting expeditions and heightened exposure to the sun. His hair, which was usually long and wispy, was cut now as dark stubble all around his head. A tiny ponytail barely touched the collar of his t-shirt, which accentuated the muscular fullness of his arms. And he wasn't wearing his glasses. Instead, his large, ebony eyes flashed animatedly from behind his long, brown lashes, and his mouth pursed seductively within his five o'clock shadow. Lori wasn't sure how much the numbing shot of intoxication through her veins was playing on her psyche that evening, but she was surprised to find herself slightly attracted to her Platonic friend of so many years.

"So to me, decorating your face with tribal war paint is completely conforming to what you think society wants," Rutherford said, smiling smugly at Angela. "You're giving in and you're selling out. That's the way I see it."

"And that's why you're alone," Angela said. Lori was just able to detect a set of piercing, defensive fangs sliding down over Angela's frosty pink lip balm covered smackers as she shot Rutherford a look of blood spraying death. "Your standards are unrealistic."

Rutherford shrugged. "To me, it just shows that a lot of girls aren't comfortable in their own skin. And instead of fighting that insecurity, they hide themselves behind something they've been brainwashed into believing makes them more attractive to a male. Now for me, it's more of a turn-on to meet a girl who isn't afraid of being herself. Who isn't afraid of being different."

Lori tilted her head toward Rutherford. "What about underarm hair?" she asked.

"Underarm hair..." he started. He moved his body back in his seat to make room for the sausage- and pepperoni-covered pizza that was placed in front of him. "Well, honestly I like a girl to shave certain areas. I don't care about a girl's legs ... But I ..."

"That is so hypocritical, Rutherford," Angela interrupted. She slapped a hot, cheese-dripping slice of pie on her plate. "A woman shouldn't lower herself by trying to enhance her looks a little, but it's vital for her to suck up to societal expectations by chopping hair off her pits?"

"It's more of a hygiene thing than an aesthetic thing," Rutherford said coolly. He bit into the tip of his pizza and began chewing with a vacant, distant look in his eyes.

"And what about you?" Angela asked, her bright blue eyes glaring beneath light patches of emerald green shadow. "What about that ... that hair cut of yours? You didn't do that to attract some attention to yourself? Some *female* attention?"

"This?" he asked, running his grease- and pizza crumb-covered fingers across his shaven head. "I did this freely. Not to prove anything to anyone. Not to get anything from anyone. Just did it. No thought. Purely spontaneous."

"But it's a style," Lori said, taking hold of Angela's arm, which was perched like a rocket ready for take-off. "You've bought into some kind of fashion meant to draw some kind of attention to yourself. Otherwise you'd be walking around like a fuzzy bearded, long-haired hobo who's under no one's influence."

"I'll probably end up going back to that look," he said, smiling at Lori.

She smiled back, and sipped some soda.

"So... You two have done it, right?" Angela asked Lori, pointing back and forth with one finger between her and Rutherford.

"What?" Lori's face contorted. She looked at Angela's wine glass, which was mostly empty. "Absolutely *not*!" She glanced quickly over at Rutherford before fixing her gaze again on Angela.

"Thanks," he said, chuckling.

"No, I mean … You know what I mean. We've never … you know. In all this time, we've just never …"

Rutherford moved his bushy brown unibrow quickly up and down and smirked at Lori.

Angela's eyes were wide and glassy. "I just … assumed that you had … I really thought you did."

Rutherford stood up then and walked behind Lori's chair. "Well at the very least, we could engage in something like this every once in a while." He began rubbing Lori's shoulders and neck very hard, so hard that she did not feel any real pleasurable sensation in them. After several minutes of getting the same tight muscles kneaded like dough, Lori felt Rutherford's hands slip away and saw him out of the corner of her eye approach Angela. She watched Angela's eyelids droop and a sleepy grin sweep over her face.

The day drew to a close.

"Bye!" Angela yelled. She hugged Lori first and then Rutherford. "We'll have to do this again, sometime!"

"Yeah, sure …" Rutherford said, patting Angela softly on the back.

They watched Angela get into her car and drive off before they headed back toward Rutherford's eleven year old Chevrolet with its corroded tire rims and dented fender. As they walked, Lori could tell by the way he was strutting alongside her that he was carrying with him a curious air of self-importance.

"So what do you think of her?" Lori asked.

"Nice," he said. "Not bad-looking, I guess."

"I think she's attractive," Lori said.

"I just think she's a little…" He paused. "Nah. Never mind."

Lori sighed. "What?"

"No, I mean, it's nothin.' She's just …"

62

"What?" Lori asked. "Lively? Animated?"

"Y-yeah... Animated ... Talkative ..."

"So what's the problem?" Lori asked.

"Nah, nothing. Look, I'd love for all of us, including your buddy there, to get together again," he said. "I'd really like that."

"This is you," Lori said, pointing to his car, which surprisingly wasn't sitting at a tilt with all of the heavy piles of rubbish filling the back seat. "What is all of that?"

"I have to clean this out at some point. I might actually have some shirts and sweaters that you'd be interested in back there. But they'd have to be washed. Possibly fumigated."

She wrapped her arms around his waist and hugged him good-bye, feeling a bizarre rush when he squeezed her tightly back. Before she could really pay close attention to what she was doing, she found herself kissing him softly, and mildly passionately, on his cheek. He looked at her for a few seconds before slowly pulling away, getting into his car, and driving silently off into the distance.

Lori headed back toward her apartment, staring hard into the concrete pavement below her feet as she staggered along. This leaning she seemed to have toward soul-less souls and Dark World entities lurking cryptically in the foreboding shadows was starting to seriously concern her. She wondered if she would ever be able to stare into the face of someone like Paul and not be simultaneously swayed by the potent mix of someone else's raging testosterone and her own undying demons.

Chapter 8

*Ordinarily he was insane, but he had lucid moments
when he was merely stupid*
Heinrich Heine (1797-1856)

From: AngelontheAirwaves3254@hotmail.com
Subject: Re:
To: LoriSolomon6697@yahoo.com
LL/SF,
I wanted to make you aware of an e-mail I got from a friend of mine ... not to depress you, but just to show you what people have gone through in this business, and how it's affected them. Tom has been in radio since the "glory days" (which are gone forever, I'm afraid). He has 30 plus years of experience, and has been fired and booted more times than God. This letter from him made me cry (literally). I think that, even not knowing him personally it will have a similar effect on you because of how sensitive you are. It's just so incredibly sad and heartbreaking, the whole damn thing.
Tom is talking about WDRR, where he worked for several years. He was the morning drive news/sidekick person. Then one day, suddenly, for no reason at all John Meyers decided to put a pretty young woman on the air (WITH NO EXPERIENCE!!!) in place of Tom. He was given the heave-ho one day, and since then has not been the same. Jesus. I don't know what to SAY to him, what to DO for him, my heart just absolutely breaks. Like he says, I may be in a good place right now, but nothing lasts in this business, it's very early in the game for me, and I should literally EXPECT to be booted at some point.
Angela

From: LoriSolomon6697@yahoo.com

Subject: Re:
To: AngelontheAirwaves3254@hotmail.com
Angela,
Your friend's got the option of making the best of what's going on in his life, or of walking around like the victim and creating more of his own problems by doing so. I'm not saying that he didn't get a raw deal. I'm just saying that people have the option of taking a bad experience and using it to actually better their lives instead of worsen it. I look at it this way. You can lie on your deathbed looking back on a life filled with struggles and defeat, but also triumph. And you can take pride in knowing you had the strength to override all the obstacles thrown your way. Or you could lie on your deathbed looking back on a life filled with anger, defeat, regret, hurt, misery, failure, and bitterness, because you never did anything to rise above the obstacles. I personally don't want to live my life like that, and I can't feel too sorry for anyone who chooses to either.
Lori

From: AngelontheAirwaves3254@hotmail.com
Subject: Re:
To: LoriSolomon6697@yahoo.com
Lori,
I agree with you for the most part. You make a lot of good points. However, I also agree with my friend Tom in many ways because I, too, have already been a VICTIM of radio corporate greed ... and this business is truly a different animal than most other businesses, DESTROYING innocent people every day. Sorry for the dramatics, but it's true. You (and I mean you personally as well as "you" generally with regard to others who are not "life-time" broadcasters) cannot possibly understand the agony unless you have "walked in our shoes."

As I said, I think you do make some good points, and I respect them. But I feel you are coming from a position of judging a "war" you have never fought. It would be like me trying to say someone who'd fought in Viet Nam should "just get over" post traumatic stress syndrome. Who am I to make that kind of judgment when I have never even been close to fighting a jungle war? I hope you can understand where I am coming from on this subject.
Angela

From: LoriSolomon6697@yahoo.com
Subject: Re:
To: AngelontheAirwaves3254@hotmail.com
Angela,
I understand what you're saying, but I think you missed the point I was trying to make. There's no arguing that Tom, and you, and anyone who's been in broadcasting have had difficult times because of the nature of the business. But I don't think wallowing in self-pity and/or spreading negativity are going to help matters. Please read more closely what I was trying to say. The self-defeatist attitude doesn't do anything but drag you and everyone around you down, and doesn't solve anything.
Lori

At least eight weeks had passed since Lori was last called into the radio station to voice commercials. The station's staff had expanded, and it seemed to be more convenient for the station's head producer to use someone in-house over Lori for weekday programming. Her only viable connection with the station had been dwindled down to sparse commercial reads for weekend hosts that she was responsible for producing on her own time. Because her internship would soon be nearing its end, she struggled to think of a way to stay connected to the station after the internship was officially over. Since the new format of the station was soon to be business, she thought of pitching the idea of reporting on the biopharmaceutical industry and bringing to light anything that might catch any miscellaneous stockholder's interest. While it would be a far cry from the fluffiness and buoyancy that had originally drawn her to radio, it would be a way of keeping her new world of broadcasting orbiting outside of her old world of science. Inspired by her brother's recent successes, she wasn't sure yet that she really wanted to completely abandon the path her brother had so nicely smoothed out ahead of her. Maybe her idea of merging her two worlds would result in her eventually having the best of both, strikingly different as they were.

Keeping her link with the radio station alive meant being faced every so often with seeing Nick, shielded behind his stone-cold and business-like daylight hours façade. She tried to avoid encountering both him and his mimed rejection by going to the station late at night when most of the staff had already left for the day. Although working late in the tiny, dark production booth near a maze of empty cubicles made Lori feel lonely at times, she knew that Nick's wild fluctuations between overt seduction and chilling indifference would make her feel even lonelier.

The image of Nick's face had stopped appearing over her car windshield as she drove through the streets of Springfield in the mornings to school. She was beginning to finally feel her attachment to him dissolve; she was able to breathe again without her heart swelling and stuffing itself in her windpipe. The time had come for her to reclaim herself, to display the proud strength of her newfound character like a beautiful grapevine-entangled pergola perched high on a hilltop and overlooking countryside meadows. She was nobody's fool; she was nobody's puppet. And she needed no validation, or closure. She was simply... unto her own.

Mostly.

"I'm just calling to make sure that you put the read I did the other night into the system," Lori said. "I left you a minidisk and a note. Did you get them?"

"And who is this?" Nick asked, playfully.

Lori paused. "Someone from your past."

"And whom might that be?" he asked.

"You know who this is."

He chuckled. "I know. I just like teasing you."

She knew she'd have to try a little harder than usual to avoid getting sucked into the depths of his multi-faceted schizophrenic malady. "It's been a long time since I've been called in to do voice-work for the station. It's also been a long time since you've called to harass me."

"Do you want me to?" he asked. "I will, if you want. I just thought that you didn't like it when I used to harass you."

"I didn't," she lied.

"Oh." He grew quiet.

She sighed heavily into the phone. "I've been writing a lot lately," she said. "It's a story of sorts, and a lot of what I've written actually pertains to you."

"Really..."

"Ah-ha. I want to make sure that you're O.K. with that."

"Read some to me," he said after a few seconds of silence.

"Are you O.K. with this?"

"Yeah," he said.

"Are you sure?" she asked.

"Yeah. Read some to me."

Lori glanced over at a tattered manila folder at the corner of her desk and picked it up. She could hear his breath hitting the receiver.

"Read to me," he repeated.

She partially lifted the folder, and then set it back down in a cloud of dust.

"So ... did you write about our ... *first time*?" he asked, slowly and suggestively.

"I glossed over it," she said. "What I'm writing is not exactly a celebration of events."

"Oh." He was quiet for a moment. "I can give you more material to write about, if you want."

"No," she sighed into the phone. "I'm really just trying ... to put everything behind me."

"That's O.K. It's all right. But just know that I'm here if you want me."

"Just make sure that you put my read into the system, O.K.?" She hung up the phone.

She recalled the vast magnetic force field surrounding him that had drawn her in time and time again. She was beginning to understand what a drug addict, alcoholic, or chronic gambler goes through when faced with that pinch of cocaine in a darkened alleyway, that sweaty bottle of Jack Daniels in a rusty toilet tank, or that lonely one-armed bandit in a crowded casino.

Nick Warren was a physical and spiritual embodiment of every boy in Lori's life that had left her longing for more. Around him she could smell the same thick, pungent odor of danger that she could sense with the rest, musky pheromones flaring her nostrils and moistening her mouth and continuing to make her crave *more*. He was her past literally coming back to haunt her. Except unlike her real past that left her feeling hollow and disillusioned, Nick teased her with the notion of finally filling that echoing void within. But this would only happen if she agreed to play by some simple rules. They were rules that didn't apply to the conventional realm she had grown to know so well, but rather to his hidden underworld of uninhibited hedonistic pleasure that she thought she would never in her waking years be exposed to. And the precise rules she had to play by simply dictated that she had to play. Period.

She wondered what drove him to want so much that seemed so meaningless in so many ways to her. Why couldn't they both lay to rest the Dance of the Macabre and settle in with each other? Didn't he like her? Didn't he want to be with her?

"Hel…loooo…" A male voice greeted Lori over the phone the following day. It was a stab at an Indian or Arabian accent.

"Nick?" she said. "Hey, look. I'm in the middle of a crisis right now and--"

"What kind of crisis?" he asked, sounding dejected.

"A pot of boiling water with noodles is overflowing onto my stove--" She stopped herself before she wasted another breath on divulging something that she figured he really didn't care anything about. "Never mind," she said, starting to lower the receiver. "I'll call you later."

"Okay. Bye."

"Bye."

Several hours passed. She drifted over to her computer terminal and began punching in her electronic mail codes with the saintliness and dedication of a missionary.

From: Lori Solomon6697@yahoo.com
nick,

i'm sorry i couldn't get back to you earlier. i tried, but you weren't in. what did you want?
lori

From: NickWarren557@hotmail.com
u

When the black, twisting, funnel of debris and condensation can be seen in the stormy distance, over fields covered by wind swept grass, sucking every living and non-living thing around it into its hungry, anarchic gut, the natural response is to run panic-stricken as far away from it as possible. Lori, for some reason, found herself running open-armed toward it, bearing gifts.

From: Lori Solomon6697@yahoo.com
in what capacity?

From: NickWarren557@hotmail.com
to have something warm

From: NickWarren557@hotmail.com
MY LAWYER IS GONNA HAVE TO READ YOUR SCRIPT, BY THE WAY... IT'S HIS DECISION TO LET YOU USE ANYTHING THAT RELATES TO ME ... 'CAUSE IF IT SELLS I WOULD BE ENTITLED TO RECEIVE SOME LARGE AMOUNT OF CASH FROM THE SALES

From: Lori Solomon6697@yahoo.com
is your lawyer the one you had to hire to bail you out when you were found in that hotel room with the five midget cross-eyed prostitutes and wild game?

From: NickWarren557@hotmail.com

MY HOES BAILED ME OUT. SO DO I GET TO HAVE
SOMETHING WARM??

From: Lori Solomon6697@yahoo.com
home-cooked meal?
blanket?
hug?

From: NickWarren557@hotmail.com
no that's not what i want

From: Lori Solomon6697@yahoo.com
you are undoubtedly the horniest person i have ever
known

From: NickWarren557@hotmail.com
SO IS THERE A PROBLEM WITH ALWAYS WILLING
AND WANTING TO HAVE SOMETHING WARM AND
WET ON ME OR NEAR ME

From: Lori Solomon6697@yahoo.com
get a puppy

From: NickWarren557@hotmail.com
well i have had your kitty before ... that felt good

Lori collapsed on her living room couch that
evening, not sure if the overwhelming fatigue she was
feeling was due to having studied long hard hours that
day, or if it was due to having tried to get any studying
done at all in between all of her e-mail exchanges. She
stared resolutely into the coffee table that sat in front of
her, trying to understand how and why it was all
happening again. The coffee table, in return, gave her
no answers, except maybe to alert her to a dust ring

around an ancient mug of cocoa that desperately needed to be washed.

She knew that she was chillingly unable to steer away from what was inevitably going to cause her a lot of pain. Having Nick Warren in her life had pinched like a sharp needle prick over and over again in the same bulging vein in the same soft region of skin. Though the puncture wounds sealed over nicely with time, the syringe was still perched and ready to take the plunge at any random point.

She had to see him early one day at the radio station, when she had organized a meeting with the program coordinator to discuss her science reports. She kept his image only in her peripheral vision, as usual, afraid that looking right at him would leave her with the same kind of regret as if she had looked directly into the stark, blinding sun.

After glancing in Lori's direction, Nick gave her a polite, yet guarded, greeting and went casually about his work. She briefly acknowledged him in return before disappearing into a small studio with the harried program coordinator. Their mutual foolproof façade was still apparently in tact, a shield of armor that in a very ironic and insidious way seemed to only add to the fragility of all that was happening between them.

From: NickWarren557@hotmail.com
i like the feeling of your ... when it gets … and when you moan a little with excitement …

From: NickWarren557@hotmail.com
i like to tease you…. lol
so what was the reason u were in today? did u get warm when you saw me?

From: Lori Solomon6697@yahoo.com
the station needs more biotech coverage. i've been getting feedback so i can do reports that will air at some point

From: NickWarren557@hotmail.com
wow that's pretty cool … you know something? I'd like to have the real thing instead of someone teasing me …

From: Lori Solomon6697@yahoo.com
i wish that what i feel i CAN give you, you'd be willing to take

From: NickWarren557@hotmail.com
and what would that be???? please tell me

Lori left the question dangling. She left it alone because she herself had no idea what she felt she could give him. She knew he had a habit of taking more than he should, and of giving less than he could. In other words, he had the ability to hurt her, as well as the tendency. And she had no idea why.

Chapter 9

Men are not prisoners of fate, but only prisoners of their own minds
Franklin D. Roosevelt (1882-1945), Pan American Day address, April 15, 1939

From: AngelontheAirwaves3254@hotmail.com
Subject: Re:
To: LoriSolomon6697@yahoo.com
Just want you to know, Rutherford and I have started a very interesting and fun dialogue. He really is a terrific guy!!! I think my initial impression of him was way off base.
Angela

From: SeriousSchmendrick4428@aol.com
Subject:
Pleeeeeeeeeeeeeeeeaaaaaaaaaaaaaaaaaaaaaaaaaaaaa sssssssssssssssse!
To: LoriSolomon6697@yahoo.com
The more I talk to Angela, the LESS I want it to turn into something. Why? Because I'm afraid that I'll actually LIKE her and that she'll ultimately find out that I'm the irresponsible, immature, and self-centered BASTARD I told you in the past that I'm well aware that I am.
Rutherford

From: AngelontheAirwaves3254@hotmail.com
Subject: Re:
To: LoriSolomon6697@yahoo.co
LL/SF,
One crucial question that I forgot to ask you about Rutherford: does he SMOKE? God, I hope not … That would be a complete turn-off. I don't even like to have friends who smoke. I know it sounds judgmental, but I

am highly allergic, plus it stinks worse than skunk or farts.
Angela

From: SeriousSchmendrick4428@aol.com
Subject: Whaaaaaaaaaaaaaa????????????????????
To: LoriSolomon6697@yahoo.com
Dearest of the Dear,
I'm really enjoying the Angela thing. In fact, I'm eagerly awaiting her next message. Weeeeeee!
Yours in Bodhisattva,
Rutherford

From: AngelontheAirwaves3254@hotmail.com
Subject: Re:
To: LoriSolomon6697@yahoo.com
LL/SF,
I've been having trouble sending e-mail. My computer has been all messed up. We NEED to talk. Rutherford and I had our first fight and we're not even going OUT!!! I'll be near the station Sunday. Let's do dinner or drinks or something.
Angela

From: AngelontheAirwaves3254@hotmail.com
Subject: Re:
To: LoriSolomon6697@yahoo.com
LL/SF,
Rutherford and I are on even keel now. We've had some great talks … and are getting together Saturday for a movie and dinner. YUM.
Angela

From: AngelontheAirwaves3254@hotmail.com
Subject: Re:

To: LoriSolomon6697@yahoo.com

Things with Rutherford and me are completely over. We might be able to be friends some day in the future, but right now we are licking our wounds. Lori, I think the guy has serious problems, and I just don't need that in my life. I tried to tell him why I could not be involved with him … and he turned the tables on me and accused me of being "pathological" for leading him on, only to crush him.

Angela

From: AngelontheAirwaves3254@hotmail.com
Subject: Re:
To: LoriSolomon6697@yahoo.com

I just wrote a long e-mail to Rutherford, detailing how his abhorrent behavior with regard to women made me sick to my stomach … and how much pain it caused me, etc. etc. Then after I sent it to him … I got an e-mail from him in response to the one I wrote last night … saying that he thought we were making a big mistake by passing up what could be something very special and wonderful. Lori, I don't know what to do!!! I am an emotional wreck right now. He is going to completely HATE me after he reads my e-mail blasting him for being an unabashedly arrogant womanizer with absolutely no respect for the female species. I even said I was grateful to the stars above that I had not succumbed to his charms and wound up in bed with him, just another wayward pussy for his collection … Oh, Lori … I am in so much pain; I have been in the bathroom going both ways eight times already. I am going to lose ten more pounds from this, which is actually a good thing, but what a way to lose it!! Help me, my friend. I am sinking fast…

Angela

From: AngelontheAirwaves3254@hotmail.com
Subject: Re:
To: LoriSolomon6697@yahoo.com

Hi, Babe,

Well, Rutherford and I had a three-hour talk last night, and straightened everything out. We both realized that neither of us is ready for a romantic relationship, but we are going to be very good friends to each other. We have a lot of "inner issues" to work on before letting someone else into our lives. Rutherford has more than I, I think, though I did not tell him that.

He is a sheep in a fox's clothing. But that "fox" can be pretty blunt and abrasive. I told him he scares me! And that falling in love with him would be hard. Do you know that he has not been "in love" since he was sixteen? With a girl named Mary who dumped him before he even felt he "had" her. He's been "playing around" since then, protecting his heart from every potential lover.

But I have been doing the same thing. And we have both built strong walls around us for protection manifested by the excess "fat" we let build up on our bodies. It's all part of the defensive shield to keep intimate relationships OUT. We have literally made ourselves undesirable physically to the opposite sex, to keep them at arm's length. It's messed up, Lori, it really is.

Angela

It was past eight on a Friday night. Lori had been asked to edit some written commercials that would be airing over the weekend, and she could have easily come in a little earlier than usual on Saturday morning to work on them. But she had been listening to the station on and off throughout the day, and she knew they had been broadcasting from a conference miles away in Stoneham. She also knew who was responsible for handling the audio equipment for live remote broadcasts, and who would most likely be revisiting the station late in the evening when she was there.

She heard the familiar sound of swooshing polyester pants growing louder from around the corridor. She looked up as Nick drew nearer to where she posed, pen in hand, heart violently pounding in her throat. She hadn't seen him in some time, and she wasn't sure how she would react upon seeing him again. She had a hunch that her feelings would be just as irrational and irritatingly intense as they had always been, and yet she knew she had to face them- and him- down at one point or another. She strained the muscles in her shoulders, stared intently down at her notebook, and swallowed hard.

"What are you doing here so late?" he asked her. He whisked his backpack over his shoulder onto his desk and set several pieces of remote broadcasting gear down on the floor.

"Working on some copy," she said languidly, feigning disinterest.

"I haven't heard from you." He migrated over to a nearby computer and sat down in front of it. "Have you been avoiding me?"

"Maybe."

"Why?"

She shrugged. "Don't know."

"Ah ..." He pretended to busy himself at the keyboard.

"I haven't heard from you either."

He continued to stare at the computer, pressing miscellaneous keys every so often. "It didn't seem like you wanted to hear from me." He turned around briefly to face her, before turning his mock attention back to the computer screen.

"So are you with anyone now?" she asked.

"Eh, there's no one in particular. It's just me. And all of them. All of them ... and me," he said, laughing.

"So have you been thinking about me?" she asked.

He nodded, smiled, and pointed to his groin. "I can't believe how quickly I get aroused around you."

A grin swept across Nick's face as he launched into a grandiose reminiscence of the unadorned intimacy they had shared over the months. He stopped talking only when someone rounded the corner from the control room and dashed in frantic haste past them toward the production studio. Nick leaned in toward the computer screen and sat as static as a plastic mannequin until the person was completely out of sight and hearing range.

"So how about we both go into the ladies' room together?" Nick said, quietly. "There doesn't even have to be any touching. You can watch me as I --"

"No," she said, softly. "I don't think so."

Nick shrugged, with a smirk on his face. He turned around to head toward the receptionist's desk in the station's waiting room. Lori followed closely behind.

A spotlight shone down from a corner of the room, casting a beam that illuminated the center of the floor. Nick fished around the darkness surrounding the cone of light for the button of the elevator that was to come and take him to street level.

"Can I have a hug?" he asked, turning to face Lori.

"Of course," she said. She draped one arm around his shoulder and the other loosely around his waist.

He sneered, "Your hand is traveling kind of low there."

"It is not," she protested. She drew away from him slightly. He lowered his head, leaned his face in toward hers, and tried to kiss her on the lips. She turned her cheek away from him and gave him a light peck, before slinking away into the darkness of the front hallway. She continued to walk silently amidst the bitter irony of the corridor's calming cream-colored walls and serene pastoral paintings.

From: SeriousSchmendrick4428@aol.com
Subject: my armpits
To: LoriSolomon6697@yahoo.com
Lori,
First I must warn you that my friend Phil is on his way here to party for the night, so I might have to cut this short before I'm finished and get back to you later.
You need to understand something about guys. Just because they can be completely divorced from emotion in relation to sexual encounters does NOT mean that they are categorically divorced from that emotion in all cases, okay? A guy may have sex with one girl and feel nothing for her, but with a different girl he could become totally emotionally attached. But yes, there are certain guys who are generally non-committal, have sex only for the sake of sex, and will manipulate girls to achieve their ends. From what you told me about that Nick guy, it's obvious that he's the type of person who doesn't have very deep emotions for anybody at all except HIMSELF, which is probably another reason why he was so attractive to you on a subconscious level. Girls are generally, and don't even think about denying it, attracted to guys who aren't exactly "nice." That's why "nice guys" almost never get any unless they have good jobs, money, or are very good-looking. My perception of girls is that you're ultimately attracted to guys who have confidence in themselves, and nobody has more confidence in himself than someone who thinks of nobody BUT himself.

As for myself, I don't know what to tell you. I think I'm kinda weird. There have been times when I've thought that I'm not really capable of "loving" anybody in the typical sense of how people describe it. As for Babette, I tell her I love her, but I definitely don't mean it. I DO feel a lot of attachment to her because of all the time we've spent together, especially traveling around the country, but as you know I could drop the whole thing without feeling all that horrible.

Think about this, too, just to give you a sense of how sinister the male mind can be. I think I'm a "decent guy." I may not "love" anyone, at least not yet, but I certainly don't want to HURT anyone. I DO have a conscience, which at times tortures me for things I have done. For example, I had an affair almost two years ago with that older married girl Pam. I haven't even SEEN her since April of two years ago, but I still keep in periodic touch with her because she's a "sure thing," you understand? Just last week I sent her an e-mail saying "I miss you" and crap like that! Do I really miss her? Hell no. I don't even LIKE her! She's got three kids with two different fathers (and guess what... the fathers are BROTHERS!). When I think of her lifestyle, I honestly get ANGRY thinking that there are people like her out there. However, she is absolutely WILD in bed; there is NOTHING she won't do or say. You see? Even though I feel nothing for her but contempt, I think about her all the time. I've looked her right in the eyes and told her I loved her before just to keep it going. And remember, you're hearing of such vile manipulation from a "decent guy" with a conscience! Just think of how mean and self-serving OTHER guys are!

Hey, Phil's here. I gotta go. I'll continue this later. Believe me I've got a lot more to say.

Rutherford (a.k.a. Una de Gato)

From: LoriSolomon6697@yahoo.com
Subject: Re:
To: SeriousSchmendrick4428@aol.com
Jesus
Lori

From: SeriousSchmendrick4428@aol.com
Subject: his armpits
To: LoriSolomon6697@yahoo.com
What was the most striking to you about what I've said so far? The fact that men are ruthless in pursuit of sex? Or the fact that I admitted to having behaved that way myself? Remember, I said I have a "conscience," dammit! I DO feel bad when I act that way, but that won't prevent it from happening in the future.
I'm sorry I didn't write yesterday, and that I don't feel like writing much now. I've been ill for the last 2 days. Dizzy and nauseous, in fact. I can't figure it out. I haven't been drinking too much or taking major drugs or anything (dammit).
I'll tell you more tomorrow. Right now my head is aching and I feel like vomiting into my shoes.
Rutherford (a.k.a. Joe Baloney)

Seven severely obsessive days passed by, with the image of Nick's face appearing in front of thunder clouds in the rainy morning sky as Lori drove to her classes, and his penetrating blue eyes closing with the setting sun at dusk as she made her way home from school. It was all too open-ended, all too unfinished, all too tempting, and all too wrong for her to continue going on as she had been. She needed to know that it was over. For only when Nick Warren was sculpted into a mere seedy memory that time could not revisit, would Lori be free. Free of the futile hold he had on her heart, free of the damaging grasp her recurring thoughts had on her mind, and free to finally send her love to where it was supposed to go.

Wherever that was.

She dialed Nick's home number one night. She wasn't entirely sure of what she wanted to say, yet hoped that perhaps she would be able to make some kind of permanent dent that would significantly change the dynamic and set them both back on the road to Spartan simplicity.

"Hello?" Nick answered.

"Hey, it's me. It's--"

"I know who it is," Nick said, a detectable edge in his voice.

"How are you?" she asked.

"Good. Good." He was rustling papers as he talked to her. "Got a lot of ... What's this? Hmmmm.... I thought I paid this."

"What?" she asked.

"No, nothing."

Silence. Stone, cold, heart-breaking silence.

"Hello?" she said.

"I'm here." He crumpled a piece of paper and must have thrown it in such a way for it to land on the floor.

"What are you doing?" she asked.

"Just going through a bunch of bills. Cleaning out house over here." He breathed into the phone as though he were heavily concentrating on something.

"So ... can ... we talk?" she asked.

"I'm all set," he said.

"Huh?"

"Where did this one come from? I thought I took care of this, too." He started breathing into the phone again. "Here are some coupons."

Lori's cheeks began to flush. Her tongue felt like the aftermath of a question mark-shaped saliva suction device at the dentist's office. She didn't know what was wrong, or why he was acting the way he was.

"You're speaking in code to me," she said. She moved her tongue against the roof of her mouth to get some moisture flowing again. "Is there someone there with you?"

"Yes," he said. He continued to hum and moan over the phone about the little annoying documents he was ferreting out and analyzing.

"So you can't talk now," Lori said.

"Not really. Why don't you call me back tomorrow night … here? That should be a good time."

"O.K." she mumbled. I guess I'll try again." She hung up the receiver.

Later that evening, one of the tires on her four year-old Subaru flattened just as she neared the exit off the thruway that would take her home. She waited impatiently as a bored, disgruntled-looking AAA representative groaned about bolts being rusted in place because the tires had never been rotated. The car was used when she had gotten it as a gift from her parents, and she figured they had taken care of that at some point. She watched the young man break out into a sweat as he struggled to remove the flat with a crank and brute force.

A feeling of loneliness swept over her. She looked up at the night sky and tried to envision how she would feel with Paul standing quietly by her side, softly patting her shoulder and giving her a gentle nod and a warm, nurturing smile. She felt uplifted for the moment, caught up in her docile fantasy. Yet when her eyes settled back on the frustrated mechanic, an echoing emptiness once again overcame her.

Lori called Nick the following day. "So who was there with you last night? A girl?"

"No!" Nick said. "No, no! Nothing like that!"

"Then who was it?"

"My mother," he said. "She was visiting me and my dad."

Lori swallowed and nodded her head, even though she knew he could not see what she was doing. "So, why did you think I called?" she asked him. "What did you think I was going to say?"

He was quiet.

"What did you think I called for?"

"I dunno."

"What? Phone sex?" she asked.

He paused. "You mean you didn't?"

She pulled the phone away from her face. "No?" she said, gently placing the phone back under her chin.

"So why *did* you call me?" he asked.

"I think we need to talk. I just really need to talk some things out with you."

There was a passage of silence. Her suggestion to have an actual conversation with words seemed to be interpreted in the same way as if she had invited him to be the target of a horse manure-throwing contest.

"So when would be a good time to get together?" she asked.

"Ummmm … I don't know."

"How about this Thursday?"

"This Thursday?" He cleared his throat, shuffled the phone between his shoulder and jaw, and sighed into the receiver. "Well … maybe. But I usually go out with friends on Thursday nights."

The temperature of her face soared. *Your friends. Of which obviously I'm not one.* She realized that he wasn't going to talk to her. He wasn't going to let her talk to him. He wasn't going to allow her to be anything other than what she had already been to him. Anything other than what he had already been to her.

A shell of a person.

He was safe so long as he didn't fully accept what was handed to him. And she supposed she was safe so long as she didn't allow herself to be taken. But she didn't understand why things had to be this way. Why were the steel armor and shields and tamper-proof safeguards there to begin with? And what would it take to get them to go away?

"Why don't you give me a call in a couple of days," he said.

"Okay."

"Bye."

"Bye."

She let those "couple of days" go by, and then a couple of days more. A full month soon blew past her, a solid four consecutive weeks of copious amounts of distance restoring an inner peace that she had not known for a good, long while. Her memory was already dimmer in just that short span of time, for he was a shell and she was a shell, and there was hardly anything tangible for her mind to hold onto. Her plan was working; her anxiety was waning, and her life was becoming her own once again.

From: SeriousSchmendrick4428@aol.com
Subject: My cat refuses to eat swordfish
To: LoriSolomon6697@yahoo.com
It's really nice out today. I want to go swimming badly, but my neighbors are all outside in their yards and I don't want them to see me with my gut hanging out. There's a guy a couple of lots over who is big and fat and he has a hairy back, but he doesn't seem to be insecure at all about walking around with no shirt on. He needs to have his back shaved. I've even thought

about jumping on top of him and holding him down and shaving his back MYSELF. Is there a law against that? The way I see it, if there's no law against fat guys with hairy backs walking around shirtless, there shouldn't be a law against shaving them against their will.
Rutherford (a.k.a. Rich Dickman)

Lori had been operating the mixing board every Sunday, killing all late night boredom and loneliness with frequent phone conversations with Helga and the creation of obscene doodles in the margins of the station's logs. Talking to Helga was at times as much pain as it was pleasure, especially when she would describe certain newfound talents under the covers, or the unique, carnal things she discovered she could do with frozen vegetables. She was swept up in her own high energy level affair that Lori had no choice but to sit back and observe, careful not to disapprove of nor condone as it was her life and her business. Yet her candidness continually served as a sort of trigger that highlighted Lori's own recent, squalid past, and her gut reaction sadly tended to be more wistful than regretful.

Lori drove into the station's lot late one evening, having been asked to assist with commercial reads for an Indian woman named Sheetal, the host of an early morning Christian talk show. It had been a while since she had visited the station in the middle of the workweek, and it felt peculiar to her. Still, she looked forward to seeing Helga, who had also been asked to voice spots for Sheetal's radio show.

She slid her Subaru in between a Silver Ford Taurus and a red Ford Thunderbird. A russet-skinned, pudgy-faced person with short, wavy black hair was sitting inside the Thunderbird on the passenger side, and Lori was having difficulty deciphering whether the individual was male or female. Even with the help of a bright fluorescent light shining down on the car from the wet leaf-filled gutter lining the roof of the building, the stranger could have just as easily been Lori's suicidal Iranian-Jewish ex-boyfriend Hank as a mustached Spanish girl named Carmelita that Lori played soccer with in eighth grade gym class. It was pouring out and almost impossible to see past the beads of water sliding down the windshield.

Lori approached the front door of the station. Her stomach lurched as Nick emerged from inside the building.

"Hey," he said. He walked sideways past her. "What are you doing here?"

"I'm supposed to meet Helga," she panted, grabbing hold of the inner door that he had just opened. "And Sheetal."

"Oh, Is Helga here? I didn't see her," he said. "Didn't see Sheetal either. Must be downstairs, those guys."

"So what are *you* doing here?" Lori asked.

"I was just dropping something off," he said, wavering in the outer doorway. He was polite, yet unnervingly edgy. "Well, I'll be seein' ya."

Lori stepped inside the front doorway and watched as Nick slid into the Thunderbird next to the mysterious entity of uncertain sexual orientation that Lori had been trying to figure out. Before his engine had a chance to fully get started, he pulled his car out of the station lot so that he and his androgenous partner could disappear fast into the dark, rain-drenched night.

A chill ran through Lori as she felt all of the same emotions come flooding forth in one fell swoop. She walked through the dusty, old hallways and began descending a stairway that led to the basement where the production work was to take place. She knew she had to keep up some semblance of composure even though she was carrying enough intertwining anxiety and desire to spontaneously combust into a puff of smoke.

Helga was in the middle of rehearsing a commercial read when Lori approached her and Sheetal. After making her appearance known, Lori quietly slipped away and crawled back up the stairs and toward the front entrance of the building. She raced out to her car to fetch her cellular phone, trying to dodge the heavy, piercing rain drops that were shooting down from the sky like soft point bullets. The rain began to tickle the top of her head as it settled into her hair. She dug her nails hard into her scalp and crouched in the damp, muddy hallway between the locked inner door and the open, outer entrance to the building. Her little tattered address book opened right to the page that had Nick's cell phone number smudged all over. She stared thoughtfully at it before dialing.

So what exactly was she planning to say to him once she succeeded in trapping him on the other end of the line? That she couldn't stand the awkwardness between them whenever they found themselves face to face, and that this was why she needed to know that it was over? Or the fact that she couldn't stand how much she stupidly ached for him whenever they found themselves face to face, and could he please tie her wrists to a couple of bed posts with some scarves and slap her repeatedly and mercilessly across the face with a whip cream-coated bull whip?

"Hello?" Nick answered.

"Hi," she said. "This is--"

"I know who this is," he interrupted. "What's up?"

"Can you talk now, or is there someone with you … again?"

"Well, I just got back home, and I'm lying here … with my girlfriend." He allowed several seconds of silence to pass before saying, "Mona and I … we both have colds."

Lori's face felt as though she had just opened a sterilizing autoclave machine with an outflow of hot, wet steam enveloping her. She knew he had been elusive for some time, but she was not prepared to hear that he was with someone else. *Exclusively* with someone else. Imagining Nick with only one mate seemed to be an unprecedented anomaly of nature, the antithesis of the free bird aura that had been proudly spiraling around him for all the months that she had known him.

"So that's … the situation," he said. He paused and allowed Lori to die a slow, painful death in the midst of deafening silence.

"I'll call you tomorrow," she said. "I still need to talk to you about something." She seemed unable to get the phone away from her lips quickly enough.

Tears welled up in her eyes, slid down the front of her cheeks, and fused with some droplets of rainwater resting on her chin. She lowered her head in her hands and raised her body just high enough to reach the station telephone.

"Yeah, Helga … I locked myself out. Could you come out here and let me back in?"

"Hold on!" Helga said, hanging up the phone.

Lori was crying when the door was opened for her.

"I just did like twenty reads," Helga said, huffing and oblivious to Lori's hysteria. "I can't seem to do this the way Sheetal wants it, and I have to go soon."

Lori nodded and kept her head bent down in an attempt to compose herself.

"What's wrong?" Helga asked. She stopped in the middle of the hallway.

"Same old problem," Lori mumbled. "Same old situation."

"I don't understand you." Helga shook her head and sighed heavily. "Why are you doing this to yourself?"

"I don't know." Lori started to sob again.

When they reached Sheetal in the downstairs production studio, Sheetal asked Lori if she could try the same commercial read that Helga had been struggling with. Lori sniffled and nodded, and watched as Helga collected her belongings and hastily walked away, obviously frustrated yet in too much of a rush to openly dwell on it.

Perhaps Lori had attempted voice-overs in the past when she was cranky or a little tired, but she had never tried voicing a script immediately after weeping hysterically. She somehow managed to gather just enough fake cheer to have her read accepted after the very first attempt, and she left the station just in time to completely fall apart in the car ride home.

From: SeriousSchmendrick4428@aol.com
Subject: Re:
To: LoriSolomon6697@yahoo.com

Angela needs therapy. I find it rather amazing how she acts like I'M the one with all the problems, while she breaks down at the drop of a hat. It's becoming rather tiresome.

I haven't showered in nearly eight days. Does that frighten you? I occasionally will dump water over my head or swab my arm pits, and once in a while I'll give my under-carriage a bit of a "how's your father?" But for the most part I have no relationship with soap in the long term. This is cool. This is real. This is IT.

Lori dialed Nick the following day. She had no pride, and no evident traces of self-esteem or self-respect. She had only a stomach that had tied itself many times over into taut knots impervious to the passage of food or drink. Robust swigs of maximum-strength Pepto Bismol were not enough to assuage her agony. The pain had started in her heart, and her gut was merely a stopover for its metastasis.

"This is the very last phone call you'll be getting from me," Lori began. She wondered if he would allow the exchange between them to go to completion, or terminate it prematurely and leave her with nothing but her unappeased anxiety. "It's just so awkward seeing you with everything that's happened."

"Yeah, I'm trying to ... push it all behind me, too," Nick said.

"Except for that one night several weeks ago," she reminded him. "When everything was resurrected."

"Yes, with the exception of that one night," he agreed.

"I can't have that kind of temptation thrown at me," she said.

"You don't have to worry about that happening again," Nick said. "There's no problem. We're cool."

Lori paused, and asked, "So are you finally settling down with someone?"

"Nah," he said.

"No?"

"Not really. I've got this kind of ... understanding with my 'girlfriend.' We can see other people if we want to," he said. "Our friends don't really understand it, but that's just the way it is."

She breathed softly into the receiver and leaned her body forward. She let a few moments of silence pass between them, and soundlessly reveled in what she sensed was a perverse kind of relief. She hung up the phone and pulled out her lab notebook and a calculator. It was definitely relief. But it was still definitely perverse. She was relieved that he was not ready to stray from his vagabond ways. Perhaps he would, some day. But for now he belonged not to one, but to many. Lori had taken to looking at relationships as being the timely union of two souls who, for a captured moment, connect with one another. This was the opposite of the Darwinian way of looking at it, in which the "bad" get weeded out and discarded and the "good" get siphoned out and cherished. She felt that so long as she seemed to be fated to a life of intense, ephemeral yet transient passion, exclusivity had no place and no purpose other than to make her feel miserable.

Chapter 10

He that plants thorns must never expect to gather roses
English Proverb

From: SeriousSchmendrick4428@aol.com
Subject: Freakin' Retaaaaaded
To: LoriSolomon6697@yahoo.com
I still don't know why you think straying from your brother's career path is "taking one hell of a chance." It ain't nuthin. Betting your whole fortune on a single roll of dice is "taking one hell of a chance," hun. What you're doing is "trying some new things." No matter what happens, I hardly see you sucking a rock-pipe in the ghetto anytime soon. Don't worry so much. Don't think so much.
Did I mention that I haven't had a beer in four days? I think I'm starting to experience beer withdrawal. Tomorrow will be a milestone, as I haven't gone five days without a beer since I was about 14 years old.
As for Angela, I just want her to GO AWAY. I haven't e-mailed her, I haven't fielded her phone calls, and frankly every time the phone has rung or wrang or rang since Sunday night I have RUN to the caller ID box to see who it is because I DON'T want to talk to her. If you see her, tell her I moved to Ecuador with my longtime gay lover Sergio.
Rutherford

From: AngelontheAirwaves3254@hotmail.com
Subject: Re:
To: LoriSolomon6697@yahoo.com
LL/SF,
I want you to know that I'm thinking of sending Rutherford a fairly scathing e-mail, giving him a big piece of my mind. I think the guy is seriously and

dangerously screwed up, and I need to tell him that. I need to ask you as a friend to please refuse to discuss this with him if he brings it up. Tell him it's between him and me, and that you want nothing to do with it. But please, Lori, I am begging you. Don't ever bring his name up with me again, and don't talk about me with him. I need you to promise me this. The only time I could tolerate hearing his name is if you decide to drop him from your life. He is poison to me, Lori, even the mention of his name. Believe it or not, he had a worse effect on me than other guys with whom I spent a much longer time. I think the reason for that is because he is so completely messed up that he has ceased to be human anymore.

So here is the last thing he wrote to me:

"Angela, I know you mean well. I really do. Do I really "need help," as you say? Well, probably, but I don't WANT it. How about if we open a dialogue here about why I NEVER had any dates when I was "Mr. Nice Guy," but now that I've got liquid nitrogen in my veins it seems like I can find women around every corner I cross, eh? Explain THAT!

Rutherford"

So Lori, here's what I really want to send to that sick, demented son of a bitch. Tell me what you think:

One of my tragic flaws involves not being able to keep my big mouth shut when I see and feel EVIL around me. And after reading this load of garbage from you, I can't help but wonder if you haven't literally gone over to "the dark side." Rutherford, you are perhaps THE most screwed-up, delusional, and downright nasty person I have ever known. There should be prison sentences for the cruel crap you pull on people. First of all, you think that being a cold-ass jerk is getting you girls. YET ... LOOK AT THE GIRLS YOU ARE GETTING, IDIOT. You're getting the BOTTOM OF THE

BLOODY BARREL, Rutherford. You represent everything I hate about your gender. You represent the worst of your gender. Yet you had the NERVE to once try to convince me that you were one of the "good guys" to whom I should give a chance. You make people like Nick Warren look like saints.

One thing that struck me the first day I met you was that you TRY so hard to be "cool," and that ALL you SUCCEED in doing is coming across like a pathetic jerk TRYING to be cool. And not REALLY cool at all. You are a fraud. A phony. A sneak, thief, and liar. You play sick mind games with people, and think that makes you a wicked cool "bad boy" to whom girls are drawn. And then, after boasting about your newfound "bad boy attractiveness" you announce that you don't WANT help!! That you don't even want to talk about it anymore. Well, SCREW YOU, you unfathomable LOSER. Screw you for wasting MY precious time trying to help your sorry ass.

Angela

From: LoriSolomon6697@yahoo.com
Subject: Re:
To: AngelontheAirwaves3254@hotmail.com
I'd reconsider sending Rutherford that e-mail. Why don't you wait until you're a little calmer? You find him irksome, bottom line. You gave him (the "friendship") a shot. I don't think he (it) deserves anymore of your energy. I would just distance myself.
Lori

From: AngelontheAirwaves3254@hotmail.com
Subject: Re:
To: LoriSolomon6697@yahoo.com
Too late. I sent it. I had to... You may hear from him after he's read it. Please back me up, Lori, as best you

can. I find him absolutely EVIL. I ended up sending him an "amended" letter, which was even worse. I am proud of what I did. Someone has to have balls enough to hit him between the eyes.
Angela

From: SeriousSchmendrick4428@aol.com
Subject: Got this friend I think you should meet
To: LoriSolomon6697@yahoo.com
So THIS is the crap I've had to deal with:
"Rutherford,
You've decided many times over to become furiously defensive with me for trying to offer input on particular issues that I'm sure you recall. You have never even had the decency to learn more about my legitimate concerns, choosing instead to berate and insult me in your usual caustic manner. This, after I was just trying to be a good, honest friend who'd made some valuable observations that she felt needed to be shared. Rest assured that I've never wanted ANYTHING from you other than a very, VERY casual friendship, at best. I would never want to be close to anyone who made me feel as badly as I did with you. I'm the type of person who tries very hard, often too hard, to see the best in people. But you are so steeped in insecurities and denial that one must wonder if you are even a human being anymore. I intend to wash my hands clean of you (and anything to do with you) after sending this e-mail. I've already wasted FAR too much of my precious time on you. I needed to say my piece, and now I have said it. But I am no longer offering you the opportunity to respond (with whatever vile thoughts you're having right now), because I am blocking you from my e-mail inbox. In closing, I am not saying you are a "bad" person, Rutherford. But I truly feel that you are in DIRE need of getting some MAJOR help for your LOSER ASS.

Angela"

From: AngelontheAirwaves3254@hotmail.com
Subject: Re:
To: LoriSolomon6697@yahoo.com
If Rutherford does bring anything regarding me up to you, you CERTAINLY have my permission (and in fact, I want you to say this) to tell him that my anger had been building up for a long time, and escalated when he ignored me. Tell him that I felt maligned and mistreated to the point where I just couldn't hold it in any longer.
Angela

From: SeriousSchmendrick4428@aol.com
Subject: Fix-ups
To: LoriSolomon6697@yahoo.com
Lori, Angela is SCREWED. She is a hateful, disoriented, immature weirdo. If you think that she was justified in ANY way in writing the things she wrote to me, then tell me now. And I promise you that I'll be shocked, and offended.
Rutherford

From: LoriSolomon6697@yahoo.com
Subject: Re:
To: SeriousSchmendrick4428@aol.com
Rutherford,
What will it take for you and Angela to realize that I don't appreciate being thrown into the center of all your madness? I think you guys really need to cool it for a while.
Lori

From: SeriousSchmendrick4428@aol.com
Subject: Weebles wobble
To: LoriSolomon6697@yahoo.com

Lori, you're absolutely right, and I apologize for getting you in the middle of crap like this. You don't deserve to have to put up with such bull. And oh yeah, you're right. Angela and I should "cool" it for a while. Like for about 30 or 40 years, maybe. Sorry again for getting you in the middle of it.

Expediently, of course,
Rutherford

Chapter 11

God gives the nuts, but he doesn't crack them
German Proverb

The slowly unfolding days and weeks should have begun to heal Lori's wounds, forming scars. Yet she continued to lick them as though they were freshly seared into her skin. She was almost completely blind to the present and only able to focus on the past, and it kept her walking backwards and stumbling into things that she otherwise might have avoided, if her eyes had only been open.

One such thing that planted itself in the midst of Lori's path was Pista Bakfark. Still not sure about changing her major to communications, she decided to do a summer internship in a *Drosophila* lab in one of the Springfield campus research facilities. It was there that she met Pista, a libidinous Hungarian M.D., who had taken temporary leave of his clinic back home to do research in the lab she was studying in. This buzzing, circling, single synapse-firing predator playfully draped itself over any and every female that dared step within the boundaries of its rather large personal space. Pista's extensive book-marked list of Internet porn on two or three of the laboratory computers, as well as his relentless lewd and inappropriate remarks, caused the laboratory head to tongue thrash him on more than one occasion behind his closed office door. Yet Pista carried on, undaunted, drinking two to four beers every night in front of still shots of fat, naked Hungarian women doing disgusting things with their private and not-so-private parts.

The hours Lori was spending in the laboratory during the weekdays stretched well into the evenings, as did Pista's. The surprisingly deep philosophical and political discussions Lori and Pista had during their late night coffee breaks were in sharp contrast to the carefree playboy image Pista had been working so hard to sustain among his colleagues. Yet it was when Lori had tried to get him to disclose his feelings about women or relationships that any hint of sobriety would fall by the wayside, and she would be faced with the same demented prepubescent antics he so promiscuously shared with everyone else.

"You are so hot," he would say to her, smiling lasciviously with his beady green eyes flashing devilishly from behind his wire-framed glasses. "I want to do you. I want to bang you so badly."

Lori had heard him say those words so many times to so many women that she barely heard him when he said them to her. She sometimes wondered if he said these ridiculous, senseless things just to keep in practice of speaking the English language, since much of the time it seemed as though there was no real thought or emotion behind any of it. Another summer intern, Marta, from Italy, would laugh off his inane propositions the same as Lori would, and the two of them ended up treating him more as an intriguing oddity than an actual person.

Lori's growing affinity toward Pista as a friend, and his growing affinity toward her, was hastened by their mutual disdain toward Pista's co-worker, Ulf Fucher, arrogant and unapproachable and far more concerned with his own professional advancement than with being at peace with his colleagues. Fucher's sociopathic ruthlessness and pathological territoriality led to the first of many anesthetically void colonoscopies that Pista would receive from him during his stay in the lab. Despite the fact that Pista eventually fell into promising work that was completely independent of Fucher's, feelings of isolation and powerlessness gave birth to a longing for an ally and a dire need for support.

From: SeriousSchmendrick4428@aol.com
Subject: taxation without representation
To: LoriSolomon6697@yahoo.com
Ulf obviously needs to get his ass TAXED. If you'd be willing, I'd be happy to tax him on behalf of your friend Pista for the meager sum of perhaps a nice bottle of olive oil and some fine cheese and a good rack of lamb. The bottom line, however, is that Ulf sounds like a positively miserable human being. He probably hates himself and everything about his own life, and is thus projecting that self-loathing onto other people. If I were a true Christian, I'd say pity him; if I were a true Buddhist, I'd say the same. However, I'm NEITHER, so I think you should kick him in the nuts and then stick your tongue out and say "Nah, nah, nah-nah, nahhhh!"
I don't know if I mentioned this to you or not, but right now I'm living in a cottage on a lake that my parents own. Last night, I made a campfire outside and sat there staring at it until about 4 AM, when I finally drained my last bottle of Wachusett Beer and stumbled inside to go to sleep. I want something bizarre and unpredictable to happen, damn it! I need action!
Why is life so god damned tedious!
It's hot and muggy here. Terrible! I have no air conditioning and no FAN either. Fortunately I DO have a lake in my back yard that I can jump into to cool off, but unfortunately I can't SLEEP in the lake. Trying to sleep in this hot muggy crap is about the worst form of torture I've ever experienced; aside from discussing politics with my sister. Did I ever tell you that I'm highly suspicious that my sister is a lesbian?
Oh well, whatever. I'm sweating bullets just from typing. I'm going to go jump in the lake, so to speak. It's late,

and it's dark, and nobody else is around... so I might even remove my shorts! Hooray!
Rutherford (a.k.a. Rutherford)

On one particularly hot and sultry summer day, Pista sat in front of a computer, brooding over a confrontation he and Ulf had just had. Lori sat down at a computer next to his and began quietly surfing the Internet.

"What happened between you guys?" she asked, peering at him out of the corner of her eye.

Pista groaned. "I don't want to talk about it," he said. He stared hard at the computer.

"What's with this friggin' thing?" Lori asked. She angrily slid her mouse over its pad and started randomly clicking on icons.

"What's the problem?"

"This stupid program. It's got all these ... kinks."

"Let me see," he said. He softly placed his large, solid hand over hers and gently guided her through the program. She felt a sudden, disquieting yearning as he did this, and she quickly withdrew her hand. Pista continued to manipulate the mouse and fix his gaze on the computer screen as though Lori had already left the room. She looked up at the clock hanging over the doorway of the office, and she rose to leave.

"See you tomorrow," she said, weakly.

"See you," he called out. He was still ogling the computer. "I squeeze your boobies," he said, absentmindedly.

Lori had to walk several blocks from the research facility to her car. A joyous smile crept across her face as she quickly darted over crosswalks, the warm, humid air massaging her neck and arms. She was feeling something very similar that night to what she had been feeling for months for Nick, except for the first time in so long, it was someone other than Nick drawing this feeling out of her. She had a strong, sweet craving for something perverse, something new. It reminded her of her need to break free from the mundane, to revitalize her soul in some way. It tapped right into the restlessness that had become so unshakably apparent in her.

But her desire seemed even more complex, borne out of a need to break through a superficial barrier, to sneak past a thin, opaque flap of absurdity and catch a glimpse of the truth. She wanted to be able to look into Pista's eyes and see the soul behind them instead of the travesty.

She slowed down her pace and soberly stared down at the darkened concrete sidewalk beneath her feet. A light mist moistened her arms and the backs of her hands and made the night air thick and heavy. She continued walking, robotically now, past an alternating display of elegant eighteenth century Gambreled homes and Georgian saltboxes, each veiled by dense shrubbery and overgrown weedy grass interrupted by purple violets and hydrangeas.

Was her curiosity about Pista as frivolous as wondering if door number three would reveal a brand-new Porsche or a cart-carrying donkey? Or did she sense in Pista a shade of the overt elusiveness of Nick? It was elusiveness that never failed to awaken the demons of mayhem deep inside her bowels. It was elusiveness that lit the fire of passion, the fire of fleeting passion.

"Dare me to?" Pista asked the following day in the lab.

"Dare you to what?" Lori asked, rhetorically, having played along with this game more times than she could remember in one sitting.

"You know," he said. He grinned at her, removed the flaps of his lab coat from his thighs and pointed toward the thin fabric that masked the great uncircumcised, Hungarian mystery that lie beneath it. "Would you like to see it?"

"See what?" She expected to call his bluff, as she had so often in the past. She stifled a yawn.

"This." He unzipped his fly and made some quick, blurry motions with his hand.

"I just saw it!" Lori said, turning her head away from him and covering her eyes with the palm of her hand.

"What?" he asked. Pista laughed nervously and tugged on his zipper. "You did?"

"Yes! I did!"

"I … I didn't mean to … I mean, I didn't think I … You did?" He stood up and started shoving his shirt into his pants. Beads of sweat glistened on his large forehead.

Lori sat in her chair, staring at him helplessly.

He walked over to her and said, "Lori! I … I … I take you out for a beer. Come. Let's go for a beer. We discuss this over a beer."

"I'm not of age," she said. "I can't order alcohol."

"It's okay. I take care of it. No one will know."

Tugging desperately at her elbow, he guided her to the local galleria where they sat down at a tall, wooden table near a restaurant bar. He smiled awkwardly at her while the waitress acquiescently fetched large glasses of Guinness.

"All right," he said, taking his first sip of beer.

"This has to stop, Pista."

"I know, I know. I am very sorry. I honestly didn't know I would … ex- expose myself."

"It's not just that," Lori said, waving her hand. "It's how … *comfortable* you've gotten around me in the lab lately. I guess that's the best way I can put it."

He nodded his head as though he knew exactly what she was talking about, and continued to drink his beer.

"You and I have gotten a lot closer over the past few weeks. You know that," she said.

He nodded again.

"All of your … moves. Like the little shoulder rubs when I'm sitting at the culture hood or the microscope. They're … they're … *getting* to me. I've been feeling kind of *uncomfortable* all of a sudden. Something's … changed."

He stopped nodding and looked into her eyes.

"I've been feeling differently around you lately. Maybe it's because we're working so closely together for such a long time. I don't know." Lori gulped some of the acrid beer down, feeling suddenly very light-headed.

"It's all right," he said.

She shook her head. "I think we've got to distance ourselves from one another a bit. You know?"

"All right." He tipped his glass back into his mouth and finished his beer.

She swallowed another quarter of her own drink, and felt a soothing peripheral numbness that made her wobble when she stood up. Guinness was one of the few beers that could lobotomize her if she drank enough of it; and very rarely because of its potency and bitter taste could she even get through a full glass of it.

They returned to the laboratory office. She felt proud of herself; proud that she could thwart desire in the face of danger. And she had faced down far too much danger in her recent past to let something as malleable as desire lead her again into its clutches. As she learned in one of her courses, in the Buddhist world desire was perceived as a standing ticket to calamity, as it could breed only attainment, which could breed only loss, which could breed only despair. Lori most certainly did not need to attain Pista, as there was nothing even remotely substantial about him to grab hold of. There was no "soul" behind his eyes, at least no soul that he would ever give Lori the chance to see. And for her to set herself up to lose mere pretense would undoubtedly brand her a fool.

Yet again.

She sat quietly in an office swivel chair, rocking herself at 30-degree angles to her left and right, staring bemusedly at a hypnotic computer screen-saver. Even if there were something more tangible there inside him, something that only she would have the privilege of touching and tasting and inhaling like no one else would dare, it was still a stopgap. No depth, no permanence, and no meaning other than a passing of the here and the now without any concern for tomorrow.

She figured she would get ready to stagger her way out of the laboratory and go home. She pushed her chair a few inches away from the computer and started to stand, when Pista swung her seat around to face him. He quickly thrust his muscular arms up through the tight elastic holding her skirt. Months of mounting tension exploded like the volcanic eruption of Mount Vesuvius as the two of them climbed drunkenly on top of one another and clawed ferociously at whatever body parts were most easily accessible. They moved as a huddled mass of entangled and partially clothed flesh into their supervisor's darkened office; two stopgaps momentarily filling a permanent void.

From: SeriousSchmendrick4428@aol.com
Subject: voy a fumar marijuana y crack cocaine
To: LoriSolomon6697@yahoo.com

God, I'm hot. It's HOT. It's muggy, too, and I've got all the windows open and there are little buggies swirling around in here like some sort of aero-bug-armada.

I've got a good one for you. My friend Jill came over yesterday with her "girlfriend" Gina. Gina was a very nice person, and pretty interesting to talk to, but I have to say that I have NEVER seen a female human being that was so completely devoid of anything feminine at all! This girl looked- I kid you not- like a 13-year old boy with a crew cut. She must have weighed about 85 pounds with not a solitary TRACE of what you'd call "breasts" or the typically shapely female "heinie." Like I said, she seemed like a great girl with a friendly attitude and everything else, but her appearance really threw me. Anyway, they were supposed to just come over for a few hours and then go back to Redhook, but they wound up staying overnight here. We bought a bunch of beer and before I knew it Jill and I were both out in the lake NEKKID while Gina stayed on the shore with her clothes on because she was too cold. Now, being in the water is one thing, but Jill kept walking up onto the shore to try and convince Gina to go swimming with us, so she'd be standing there totally naked by the light of a campfire and all I could do was hover in the water with my engorged weenie sticking up through the surface like some kind of obscene periscope. It was really kind of funny, if not annoying. I mean, there's Jill standing on the lawn naked with her big breasts hanging down and ME in the water with my phallous harder than titanium alloy and all Jill is interested in is pleading with her androgynous "other" to come join us. They went to bed shortly after that, and I stayed out by the fire trying to focus my concentration on Mickey Mantle or Pedro Martinez so I could finally soften up enough to be able to put my shorts back on without breaking my Johnson in half.

I'll let you go. My friends gave me these odd little pills that they said would "mellow me out." If I get any "mellower" I'm going to wake up three hours from now with my face pressed into this keyboard and QWERT pressed into my left cheek. I'll talk to you later.
Rutherford (a.k.a. Crafty Lombardo)

Pista had decided to leave the lab within weeks of a Chernobyl-like radioactive spill that contaminated the entire laboratory as well as surrounding rooms and three quarters of the adjacent hallway leading to the departmental elevators. He stood admiringly in the doorway of one of the sullied rooms, watching Lori as she kneeled over a screeching Geiger counter with sneakers covered in blue, disposable slippers. She sulked while she scoured a ^{32}P -covered floor with paper towels saturated with distilled water and detergent.
"Could you ... come here?" Pista asked
"Huh?" Lori looked up at him, dizzy and nauseous. She threw a soaked pile of radioactive towels into a plexi-glass container and carefully removed her latex gloves from her hands. She gently peeled off her slippers and tossed them in the trash as well, before tiptoeing across what she hoped was a clean patch of floor toward Pista.
He pulled her into the laboratory office from the hallway, turned off the light, and hugged her so tightly that she was lifted several inches off of the boarded-up, still-radioactive floor. He kissed her hard on her lips and squeezed her again until she could not breathe.
She stood, paralyzed in his tight clutches. She didn't know quite what to make of his sudden fervor, but decided at long last not to think too much about it. After all, it would be gone, and he would be gone, well before

the last trace of spilled ^{32}P, with its several week half-life, disintegrated to mere background level counts.

Lori pictured herself as a flame that flickers on a dying wick for a while and eventually burns itself out. And this would not be such a bad thing if she could just learn to enjoy the brightness and heat of the fire while it lasted. But she longed for a flame that was eternal. And there just didn't seem to be nearly enough fuel to fire a passion that would last. At least not in Lori's world.

Chapter 12

Better to light a candle than to curse the darkness
Chinese Proverb

From: SeriousSchmendrick4428@aol.com
Subject: Duck!
To: LoriSolomon6697@yahoo.com
Dearest,
I dropped Babette off at the airport this morning. It was great to have sex constantly for the last week, but things between us took a drastic change last night. I'm still in a state of near-shock about it, because it confirmed some things that I've wondered about myself, and it brought home some very important points that I need to deal with.
Basically, we started talking about the whole "us" thing. She brought up the subject. In a nutshell, she told me that she feels like I've "used" her, treated her like an "object," and that I'm "selfish, cold, calculating, manipulative," and that I have "little or no conscience" about other people's feelings. She basically described ME as the same person that I've told you that Nick is, even though I don't know the guy! I was like "Okay ... I see your point ... NOT!" I told her that I was sorry she felt that way, and that I'm the type of person that has a hard time letting my feelings show, and that I really do have a conscience about things. God dammit ... the mere fact that I can't bring myself to tell her that I don't want to see her anymore is proof that I DO have a conscience and that I DO care about peoples' feelings, isn't it!?!?
Who knows? I've drank a pint of Stolichnaya and six beers in the last couple of hours, so I'd better get outta here before I start rambling about stupid crap.
Yours in the madness of life,

There was something deep inside of Lori that was still crying out for the development of some kind of connection, or disconnection. Whatever it was that was squirming around inside of her, it seemed to be aching for answers to as-of-yet unasked questions. She supposed she had many inner voices screaming to be heard, voices of the sort one would hear in a padded room in Bellevue.

She hadn't heard from Nick for quite some time. It had been months since he had scooped up the ball that had landed in his court after the seemingly endless push-pull battle of the egos. It had been months since she had succumbed to his overtures, out of a weakness she could not explain, and he had run away to leave her behind in a nebulous cloud. And it had been months during which she realized that she needed to treat him like a particle- and ray-emitting radioactive substance in the laboratory, and minimize her exposure by increasing her distance, and decreasing her time.

Then she saw him. He was filling in for one of the board operators in the station's control room, and was taking a break at his desk when she approached him. She gave him a quick nod, and continued onward toward a secluded, soundproof studio. She said nothing to him, and he said nothing to her. They did not even look directly at one another. Yet simple peripheral glimpses of him out of the corner of her eye resurfaced an old familiar unsettling preoccupation. The little intimations of his presence, salient reminders of his existence, both saddened and frustrated her at the same time.

The autumn sky harbored a full moon, a tremendous pale yellow circle, unmistakable behind two dark branches outside Lori's window. She sat perched over her computer, wondering if the lunar roundness and the oddity it was supposed to invoke would help or hinder her thoughts.

She felt a stabbing pain as her eyes fell upon some old messages of Nick's, still left undeleted among hundreds of miscellaneous messages she had never found time to remove from her e-mail site. After such a long span of time of not seeing or talking to him, his essence had reappeared for a second time in one day. It was just as real or surreal as any of the other hundreds of type-written messages he had personally sent to Lori over the past year. Seeing something that belonged to him on her computer screen was as nostalgic as smelling the scent of a fragrance she had used the night of her senior prom. It was sadly intoxicating.

Still, there was a dormant anger that began to well up inside of her at the sight of his name. It poked and prodded at her, and formed little bumps that raised the light hairs on the surface of her arms.

The full moon sprayed its black magic. Lori's fingers began dancing on the computer keyboard and transformed her into an anonymous entity, an entity primed to experience the unlimited possibilities that could arise from being camouflaged. She could become invisible, and yet ever so apparent all at the same time. It was a notion that fed into her like a delightfully decadent banana split sundae on a scorching hot Sunday afternoon.

"Desiree Jones" became her cyberspace alter ego. The name had popped into her head because of someone she had known in high school. The real Desiree Jones had been a beautiful Afro-American girl with big, soulful eyes and rich chocolate skin, and what always looked like a hint of a smile on her face. She had radiated elegance and a confidence that Lori always secretly admired, and also silently envied. Now Lori wanted Desiree to say all the things she so badly wanted to say yet had been unable to. She wanted Desiree to go on journeys that she didn't have the daring to go on herself. She wanted Desiree to disassemble the thick, shiny armor that hid the vulnerable, human side of the boy that Lori was never able to expose on her own. She wanted Nick, for once, to feel and be as vulnerable as he had made her feel and be for so long.

From: Desiree Jones
A friend of mine told me about you. She said you were good. Is this true?

 With one eye open and the other sealed shut, she stared at the words "message sent." It was done, and she calmly shut down her computer. Yet sickly warmth slowly started filling her cheeks and creeping up her neck. Suddenly she just wasn't sure how much she really wanted to connect with him again. She had been holding her own for such a long time, nurturing herself, succeeding in breaking free from his hold. After having come so close to emancipation, why would she opt again for imprisonment?

 She woke up the next morning and logged into her e-mail. She saw the number "1" in the "unread messages" slot.
 It was indeed a message.
 It was from NickWarren557@hotmail.com.
 Contact had been made.

From: NickWarren557@hotmail.com
well it depends on who is asking!!!

From: Desiree Jones
Who do you want to be asking?

From: NickWarren557@hotmail.com
first of all, a nice attractive female.

There was a familiar comfort in watching the resurrection of something Lori believed had ended. And yet, knowing that the resurrection was tainted by deception and fueled by a kind of psychotic vengeance made her feel ashamed. While she had no great love for being wounded, it was easier for her to live with the pain of her own war borne contusions than it was for her to bear the sight of those she knowingly inflicted on someone else.

Desiree Jones had to be defused. She would never bring any kind of closure to the silent humiliation that had been left lingering in the stale air. All that remained was the risk of her secret being revealed. Too much of anything in life was too much indeed. But before Desiree could vanish like she never existed back into the mysterious cyberspace from which she came, Nick started to send inquisitive messages to her. At least for the moment, it looked as though the lie had been believed, the bait eaten by the fish, the wild fowl attracted to the decoy.

From: NickWarren557@hotmail.com
I WAS JUST WONDERING... who mentioned me to you???

From: Desiree Jones
Someone you had a really good time with. Feel free to guess, if you want.

The interaction ended there. She assumed he had left for the day. She logged off the computer and started to work on some Calculus problems at her desk. She blankly stared down at a page of notes. *Pythagorean theorem. Limit of differentials. Arc length. Inverse functions.* The words meant nothing to her as thoughts about her new connection were oversaturating her mind. Where was it to go? He sounded accessible, curious.

He also sounded vulnerable.

She was excited about the prospects. As long as she kept the mystery alive, perhaps it was possible for her to keep the connection alive as well. The question was, did she want a connection with him that would last indefinitely? More importantly, did she want the kind of connection that was based solely on fantasy? Was he capable of relating to someone for the long-term in any way *other* than as a fantasy?

Was she?

It was late, and Lori was in bed. She pulled the covers over the bridge of her nose and stared up at little bumps of splattered white paint on the surface of an otherwise smooth ceiling. Keeping every inch of herself warm and sheathed in her blanket, she closed her eyes and tried to fall asleep. Yet there was too much emotion circulating inside of her; too much confused energy rebounding within the walls of her body like a bouncing silver sphere in a pinball machine.

Nowadays, there seemed to be an unlimited number of games people could play with each other, almost fearlessly, in unnerving silence. The Internet was a soundproof room within which anyone could scream anything they wanted to on the top of their lungs, with no one on the outside to hear. And even on the inside, the identities of the screamers were protected by a maze of walls, some higher than others, some lower. There were instant messenger "privacy preferences," giving you control over who could see you and who could not, who could contact you and who could not. There were ways to block e-mail addresses and prevent mail from coming through from certain people you did not want to hear from. All had the same protective purpose; all had the same ability to allow some in, to shut others out. And all had the same underlying intent: to facilitate communication, but to destroy intimacy.

From: NickWarren557@hotmail.com
joyce,
sheri,
mona,
jenn
am i close????

From: Desiree Jones
No

The discovery of things that you did not, in reality, wish to know, was one of the ramifications of posing as one's own private emissary. Lori realized then that *she* was vulnerable as well. Perhaps she was even more vulnerable than Nick was.

From: NickWarren557@hotmail.com
what about kerry, julie or misty??
i've been so good for so long that i can't keep up with all their names ☺
so just tell me who said all that stuff to you!!!!!

From: Desiree Jones

No

From: NickWarren557@hotmail.com
so why are you messing with me???? why wont you just tell me?? so what is your point in emailing me?
so what is in it for me or you with all these emails????

From: Desiree Jones
I heard you were good. I wanted to find out for myself. Are you available?

From: NickWarren557@hotmail.com
ok … so what is the next step you want to take?
how do i know you are telling the truth? how do i know if you are a female???

From: Desiree Jones
How many guys do you know that are named Desiree? And you didn't answer my question about availability. What's your situation?

From: NickWarren557@hotmail.com
WELL I'LL TELL YOU THAT WHEN YOU TELL ME MORE ABOUT YOU OR WHO TOLD YOU ABOUT ME

From: NickWarren557@hotmail.com
MAYBE SOME ONE IS MESSIN WITH ME

From: Desiree Jones
No one's messing with you. You've got my name. What else do you want to know?

From: NickWarren557@hotmail.com
WELL I WOULD LIKE TO KNOW WHO MENTIONED ME TO YOU? NOT TO BE MAD AT THEM OR ANYTHING LIKE THAT. JUST WONDERING

From: Desiree Jones
I don't want to say.
Are you still in touch with any of the girls you mentioned?

From: NickWarren557@hotmail.com
NO I WAS JUST NAMING SOME OF MY FRIENDS. SO WHERE ARE YOU FROM?

From: Desiree Jones
My friend met you in Belchertown

From: NickWarren557@hotmail.com
ok now we are getting closer … so if you trust me you will tell me who told you about me … i won't say a word … i'm just getting boggled here thinking of who told you ... please tell me!!!!

From: NickWarren557@hotmail.com
SO LET'S SEE…. BELCHERTOWN.
COULD THE PERSON BE BRENDA OR LORI?

From: Desiree Jones
Are you interested in getting to know me, or do you only care about who told me about you?

From: NickWarren557@hotmail.com
WELL YEAH I WOULD LIKE TO GET TO KNOW YOU, BUT WILL YOU EVER TELL ME WHO TOLD YOU ABOUT ME?

From: Desiree Jones
Let's get back to you. Tell me about yourself.

The exchange abruptly ended. After several moments, Lori logged out of Desiree's site and shut the computer down. She was convinced that people were turning into cyborgs, their brains governed by modern world cybernetics, a mini universe with endless possibilities. They could be actors or actresses incognito; they could get their hearts thumping fiercely in their chests without moving from their seats. She marveled at how easy it was to hide from others, and at the same time how easy it was to reach out. Life for her seemed to be becoming a sort of virtual reality with virtual relationships. Progressive technology had created a venue where the lonely could go to ease their suffering without risk. All the same, she wondered if perhaps it wasn't progressive technology that had contributed to the loneliness in the first place.

From: SeriousSchmendrick4428@aol.com
Subject: Rug burn
To: LoriSolomon6697@yahoo.com
Dearest,
Babette called me yesterday. Oh boy was it fun. Once again, she tells me I'm a "manipulator" and that I'm just "using" her. I was like "Okay... so what do you want to do about it?" I thought she'd tell me to get lost, but NO! She quickly softened up and before I knew it she was making plans for us to get together and drive up to Oregon in March.
Lori, the bottom line here is that I don't think I'm "manipulating" anyone. If she wants to send me money or buy me an airline ticket to Kansas City even though I did NOT ask for it, does that make me a "manipulator?" HUH? The only reason I said I'd like to go to Oregon with her is because I didn't want to hurt her feelings!!!! I'm not "manipulating" anyone!!!!! I don't even WANT to go to Oregon!!!

Manipulate THIS!
Rutherford Gimby

Lori had been sitting upright in her bed for hours, keeping one eye on a paperback novel, and the other on the fragmented numbers flipping over on her digital clock. She closed her book and threw it on the floor. She turned the light out, and her ears filled with the same thick silence she heard every night shortly before falling asleep. She let the echoes of emptiness lull her into a light, restless slumber tainted with a cautious anticipation of what the following day would bring.

From: NickWarren557@hotmail.com
YOU WANT TO KNOW ABOUT ME. WORK FOR AN AM DADIO STATION IN BELCHERTOWN. THAT KEEPS ME BUSY. SO WHAT DO YOU LOOK LIKE AND I JUST WONDERED WHY YOU WOULD TAKE SOMEONE'S WORD ON HOW "GOOD" I AM?

From: Desiree Jones
AM dadio station?

From: NickWarren557@hotmail.com
AM radio station

From: Desiree Jones
What kinds of looks or personality turn you on?

From: NickWarren557@hotmail.com
TELL ME WHY YOU ARE SO INTERESTED IN ME?? HOW CAN YOUR FRIEND'S WORD BE SO STRONG THAT YOU WANT TO KNOW MORE OF ME

From: Desiree Jones
What type of girl are you attracted to???

From: NickWarren557@hotmail.com
a lot of different things in a girl turn me on … the hair, the eyes, the body, the way she acts, and also the little things she does.
what's your number so we can talk more?

From: Desiree Jones
I'd like to get to know you better this way first.
You leave early, don't you?

From: NickWarren557@hotmail.com
no i don't leave early … i leave around 5-ish … so what part of the story that your friend mentioned really got you turned on to me? where did i meet your friend in Belchertown? you sound pretty mysterious, that's got me in a confused state right now!!!!

From: NickWarren557@hotmail.com
hey by the way what kind of guy turns you on? you haven't mentioned much about yourself. if your friend knows me then she must have told you more about me than i have already told you.

    Another session ended for the day, and this time Lori was the one to walk away from it. She knew she would be in store for another restive night. More pulses of energy would shoot around her insides. Synaptic explosions would ripple through the muscles of her arms and legs and cause her to mold her bed sheets into damp, sweaty twists.
    From behind closed eyelids, late at night, she could see clouds moving swiftly across the sky and dark patches of emptiness emerging from behind them. If there were distant stars that were out of scope, she

would never know. For all she could see were the clouds, and the emptiness.

From: Desiree Jones
What experiences stand out most in your mind? Who in your past really made you feel GOOD?

From: NickWarren557@hotmail.com
i'm open to trying lots of things……. what do you have in mind that we do? try some really exciting???

From: NickWarren557@hotmail.com
i'm open to trying lots of things….. what do you have in mind that we do? try some really exciting???

From: NickWarren557@hotmail.com
i'm open to trying lots of things … what do you have in mind that we do? try some really exciting???

From: Desiree Jones
Didn't I get this message already?

From: NickWarren557@hotmail.com
i sent it only once

From: Desiree Jones
Well I received it three times. See? You 're so good at giving it you don't even realize it when you are

From: NickWarren557@hotmail.com
hehe ... you should try me

From: NickWarren557@hotmail.com
so when are you gonna give me your number so we can hook up??????

From: Desiree Jones
I am someone you know.
Are you surprised?

From: NickWarren557@hotmail.com
yeah, so give me some more hints!!!!!!!!

From: NickWarren557@hotmail.com
i'm busy here at work and thinking of a million things at
once
ok here's my guess
sheri
heather
hope
jenn
pam
kelly-jo

From: NickWarren557@hotmail.com
so am i right on any of those guesses??????

From: Desiree Jones
Forget it

From: NickWarren557@hotmail.com
could this be Lori???

From: NickWarren557@hotmail.com
why should i forget it?????? tell me

She walked away from the computer. Her body
was vibrating, mildly convulsing with each wave of
bedlam that swam underneath the surface of her skin.
She walked into her bathroom, turned on the shower,
and dunked her head under a spray of lukewarm water.
When she emerged, her hair tucked messily under a

towel, she noticed that the red voice-mail message light was glowing on her phone. She pushed numbers to retrieve the message so quickly that the automated female voice-mail operator claimed she did not understand the code. Lori tried again, more slowly, her sweaty fingers slipping off of the edges of the buttons. She impatiently waited to hear what had been left for her.

"Hey, Lori. It's Nick. Here at work." His voice had a sardonic tone. "Give me a call at the station. Just gonna ask you a quick question. Bye."

She swallowed hard. Instead of calling him back, she quietly returned to her computer. She logged back onto her e-mail.

From: NickWarren557@hotmail.com
SO WHY DID YOU DO THIS?

From: NickWarren557@hotmail.com
SO YOU NEED MY SERVICES

From: NickWarren557@hotmail.com
SO YOU SHOULD HAVE LET ME KNOW AT THE STATION LAST SATURDAY. I WOULD HAVE SATISFIED YOUR NEEDS TO THE EXTREME.

From: NickWarren557@hotmail.com
so why no response???? huh?

Chapter 13

Friends may come and go, but enemies accumulate
Thomas Jones (1892-1969)

Days of aimless seduction and deception had suddenly come to a screeching halt, and Lori found herself unprepared to deal with her exposure. She was having such difficulty justifying her actions to herself, how could she possibly explain her behavior to another? She had tried to get faceless words on a computer screen to provide clues as to how he was feeling, *if* he was feeling, what he was thinking. She had tried connecting with him through the guise of a stranger, simply because she had failed to make this connection on her own. Yet why it was so important to sneak a taste of his forbidden fruit seemed to be an even bigger enigma to her than the truth of who he really was.

She knew that no intrinsic good could come of accepting the overtures she herself had made. He was a flesh-nibbling carnivore lurking in the shadows of a blood-splashed den. And she had made herself prey. It was as simple as that.

Her phone was ringing.

"Hey, there," Nick said, stretching out the lengths of his words.

"Hey."

"So?" he asked. "What was all that for? Huh?"

"Not sure," she breathed into the receiver. "I guess I … I don't know."

"What? Tell me."

Silence.

"Please?" he begged. "Please tell me."

"I ... wasn't sure if ... if you still wanted me, or not."

"I want you," he said.

"Really?"

"Yeah."

"So ... do you ... want to get together ... sometime?" she asked.

"Yeah."

"When?"

"How 'bout next week?"

"O.K." she said.

"O.K." Pause.

"All right." Pause. "Bye."

"Bye."

From: Desiree Jones
Tonight?

From: NickWarren557@hotmail.com
ill be at the station til sign off!!!!!! tonight

Lori's phone rang. She raced to answer it.

"Did you get my e-mail?" Nick panted into the receiver.

"I just got it a second ago," Lori said.

"So you wanna come by tonight?"

She paused. "There's an errand I have to run, but after that I'm free."

"O.K. Could you drive me to my car afterward? It's at the Commuter Rail."

"Sure."

"O.K."

"Bye."

"Bye." He quickly hung up the phone.

Lori arrived at the deserted station to find Nick looking harried and tired, with his taut mouth positioned in a straight line across his face, his body rigid and mechanical. It was obvious that there was some place else he wanted to be, yet he dutifully followed her into the rear, dimly lit production studio and immediately began going through motions like an actor in a XXX feature film.

"You can leave those on," he said, pointing down to the woolen socks she had started to slip off of her feet. "You don't need to unbutton your blouse, either."

She stood awkwardly near him, not understanding what, if anything, he wanted from her that evening. As he started moving his hands and pelvis thoughtlessly about, she stupidly followed his lead.

He leaned against the wall of the studio. He placed his hand on his sweaty forehead and gazed distantly at her.

"You all right?" she asked.

"Yeah," he said, solemnly. "I didn't eat anything all day, and I just got dizzy for a second."

They merged again, two dogs in heat barking orders and changing positions many times over in a crowded recording studio in the back of a dark, vacant radio station. For the next twenty minutes, Lori was a rubber blow-up doll, an inhuman porno shop sex toy prodded and bent by someone who was barely aware that she was even there.

"Would you ... like to get together again sometime?" Lori asked as she drove him to his parked car at the Commuter Rail train station several towns away. She knew that if his behavior had been any different that evening, there would be no need for her to ask him such a question. She also knew that if his behavior had been any different, there would be no need for her to ask herself the same.

"Mmmm ... possibly," he said, with a hint of a smile on his face. He grew quiet as she drove along the highway. He turned his head briskly away from her.

"Is there anything wrong?" she asked. His stillness bothered her. There was evident anger in his eyes as he gazed out the passenger side window.

"I dunno," he said.

They drove along in silence for quite some time. She cleared her throat and looked over at him. He was still staring out the window at the passing, darkened landscape.

"What's wrong?" she asked.

"I dunno," he said again.

She knew that he hadn't eaten, and wondered if it was just his hunger that was making him irritable. After all, he had seemed fine earlier in the day.

He shifted uncomfortably in his seat and continued watching a blur of black trees sweep by. "Sometimes, I feel ... guilty, I guess, 'cause of Mona."

A deafening hush that lasted through several traffic lights and a well-illuminated bridge made Lori feel queasy. Her palms were so clammy that she was having difficulty gripping the slippery steering wheel, and her mouth and throat had become so dry that she couldn't swallow without needing to cough.

In a weakened, hoarse voice, she made a desperate attempt to ease the tension, to make some sense out of what had quickly become so senseless. "So ... tell me a little about yourself," she said.

"There's *nothing* ... that you need to know about me," he growled.

Alas, he had somehow over the course of the night transformed himself into a salivating, crimson-eyed, bat-like creature from the deepest recesses of the most sinful compartment of Hell. Like a released coiled spring, the excruciating silence came back and lingered hatefully in the air until Nick reluctantly sliced through it.

"Hope wanted to get together with me a couple of weeks ago," he said. "And I ended up canceling out on her."

Hope was someone Nick had met long ago through the Internet, an Asian girl whom he had boasted many times about to Lori at the Belchertown station. His relationship with Hope had always been strictly sexual, and he claimed that neither had wanted anymore from the other than that. Lori said nothing in response, not sure if he was trying to make her feel better or worse, or if he was just trying to fill the achingly abundant stretch of time ahead of them.

"Then why did you invite *me* out to see you tonight?" she asked.

"I don't know," he said, casually. "I guess it was the messages ... that got me going. I really don't know." He stared hard at an overhead telephone wire lining the road.

She sat statuesque in her seat. The mix of songs that she was playing off of an old homemade cassette transitioned from carefully cued up classic rock masterpieces to one-hit ninety wonders that she had forgotten she had once liked. The nasty music was feeding far too fittingly into the humility of the moment. She started to move her hand toward the fast-forward button on the stereo, yet the impenetrable force field that seemed to be surrounding Nick blocked her from getting anywhere in and around the passenger seat he sat brooding in. She pulled her arm back and impatiently waited for the music to end on its own.

Nick began talking again. Lori listened semi-attentively as he described his fantasy of getting bisexual Mona together with sexually liberated Hope and watching from a short distance as they performed for him. She listened, digested, absorbed, and stifled her tears just long enough for the two of them to finally reach the train station. He closed the passenger side door without saying another word to her, walked swiftly away to his car, and left her alone.

The following morning, Lori struggled to get out of bed. She sat down in front of the computer, and stared blankly at her e-mail "inbox." She opened an old, unread message that Rutherford had sent to her the day before. Her eyes heedlessly glossed over each line, taking in each typed word but failing to grasp any attached meanings.

From: SeriousSchmendrick4428@aol.com
Subject: Bun fun
To: LoriSolomon6697@yahoo.com
I swear, chilly nights like these here at the lake make me honestly feel like despite all the crap in life I really am the luckiest son of a bitch in the world. I LIKE being alone here with my cat and the natural order all around me. It would be nice if I had an 18 year-old Swedish cheerleader waiting for me in the bedroom, but I can't ask for TOO much, eh?
I feel inspired. Let's write a play, Lori. We could be like Shakespeare. Anon, good lady! Were I to know thy breath but for a night then may the devil take me in the morning!
Piz-eace!
Rutherford

Lori clicked the mouse of the computer and exited her e-mail site. She noticed that the little glowing red light on the phone by her desk was on. She had turned the ringer off the night before, and so wouldn't have known if anyone had tried calling her. She forced herself to listen to a message that had been left on her voice-mail.

"Lesbian lover!"

It was Angela's voice.

"It's like two in the morning, and I just wanted to let you know how much you've come to mean to me as a friend, even though we've really only known each other a short time. I know this message sounds horny ... Oops! I said 'horny'!" She giggled. "I was going to say either corny or hokey, and it came out as... horny! Isn't that hilarious? I crack myself up sometimes."

Lori slowly placed the receiver down and sighed heavily. She was so far gone that she could only see darkness, even in the glow of blinding light. She lifted the receiver of the phone back up and began dialing.

"Hello?" Nick said in a cheery voice.

"This is Lori."

"Oh, hi," he said, his tone deepening.

"Are you upset with me?" she asked. "You seemed so … *angry* last night."

"No," he said, laughing lightly. "No, I'm not angry at you. I was just … really tired."

Lori could barely hear him over the fulminating sound of her own thoughts. The words, "What we did last night was so, so wrong, and I'm so, so sorry," fell from her lips and into the receiver before she could really comprehend what she was even saying to him. "I've never hated myself more than I do now." She felt that the words she had chosen sounded embarrassingly familiar, as though they had snuck into her memory from an old Grade B movie.

He was quiet for a few seconds. "Well … um … Thank you for calling. And I'll talk to you soon, O.K.?"

"Good-bye," she said. She hung up the phone in the same automated way that she had lifted it. She walked back over to her bed, sat down on its edge, and then slowly leaned her back against the mattress. She pulled the covers up to her chin. It felt as though a love affair had ended, except her anguish this time around was compounded by the guilt of knowing it never should have been, and the humiliation of recognizing that it barely even was.

Chapter 14

How much more grievous are the consequences of anger than the causes of it
Marcus Aurelius (121-180)

From: SeriousSchmendrick4428@aol.com
Subject: Da Regulatah
To: LoriSolomon6697@yahoo.com
Dear Lori,
Lord, I miss you. I just realized that it's been 12 days since we exchanged any messages, which I think is by far the longest time since we started this computer relation. I apologize for that. I don't know why I've been in such a reclusive zone for so long, but I think some of it has to do with the fact that my roommate is a bit of a nosey bastard, so every time I'm doing anything on this computer he's looking over my shoulder saying "Whatcha doin? Who are you writing to?" And I LIKE the guy too much to say "Hey... PISS OFF! It's PERSONAL!" That's no excuse, actually. I guess it's because I've been having bizarre mood-swings lately... like sometimes I'm all zippy-wippy and optimistic, but most of the rest of the time I'm just frustrated and pissy-wissy and I don't feel like doing anything except drink beer and smoke weed and listen to very loud music with my headphones on. I'm lost in a zone of meager employment, a small circle of good friends, and a demonic propensity for self-annihilation. Wow! That was a pretty cool sentence, eh? Jesus ... I wish I had something interesting to say, but I don't. The only thing on my mind right now is that I wish I had some chocolate milk and a couple of twinkies, believe it or not, but I'd rather not confront my complete apathy for existence by indulging in fat and calories. Twinkies are

awesome, though, aren't they? And chocolate milk doesn't suck either.

I'm gonna get out of here. Let me know what's happening with you and your classes and all that. Even though it's only been a couple of weeks since we "spoke," I feel like you're slipping AWAY, which is largely my own fault, of course, but it still bugs me. I'm having Lori withdrawals. It's kind of like delirium tremors, but without the fever and the shakes and the anxiety and the massive auditory and visual hallucinations. We should at least TRY to make plans to hang out or at least talk on the phone sometime, regardless of how microcosmic the odds are of that actually happening.

I'm outta here. I need CHEESE.

Rutherford (a.k.a. Francesco de brebis au lait cru)

"So Lori," Angela began. Her tone of voice over the phone was serious, yet in somewhat of a somber way. "This'll make you feel better. *A lot* better…"

"What?" Lori asked, hesitantly. She felt that there was very little at this point that could be offered to her in the form of uplift or support, except perhaps a very expensive and stylish Victoria Secret's padded bra.

"I was doing my midday newscast when Nick was running the board, and I got the chance to talk to him over the line feeds. First of all, his girlfriend left him."

"Huh?" Lori was startled by the strange turn of events in light of everything that she had experienced.

"His girlfriend apparently had had enough and walked out on him. And the ridiculous thing was that I had to *ask* him about her first, before he said … almost as an *afterthought*, Lori, something like, 'Oh yeah… we broke up.' Can you believe that? He was *living* with her, and his attitude was like, 'here today, gone tomorrow, oh well.'"

"Huh," Lori said, only able to utter caveman-like grunts of acknowledgement. She was weak and numb from her steady liquid Ensure diet and her depression, and Angela's intensity seemed to be more than enough to sustain the two of them throughout the conversation.

"So I asked him if he would miss her. And you know what he said?"

"What?"

"He said something like, 'the one thing I'll miss will be not being able to *get some* anytime I want!' Can you believe him? He *lived* with her!"

"Jesus," Lori said, hoping that she could help enrich the soul-less overtones of the situation by bringing some religion into the picture, even if it wasn't *her* religion per se.

Angela went on. "So I asked him how he could be so *cold* about all of it. And do you know what his response was?"

"What?"

"He said, 'Look, this is the way I am. This is the way I always have been, and always will be. If 'they' can't accept that, then it's out of my hands. I can't help it if 'they' get hung up on me.' Do you *believe* the arrogance?"

"Hmmm," Lori said.

Angela continued. "He said, 'I refuse to let my heart get in the way, I refuse to get attached because I don't wanna get hurt.'" Angela paused to take a deep, overly-excited breath. "So I said, 'Nick. How old are you? You're twenty-one? You sound more like a thirteen year-old!'"

"Huh," Lori said, somewhat intrigued, yet not sure she completely understood Nick's reasons for being as noncommittal as he was coming across. Was it really just profound immaturity?

"Then I said, 'And what about Lori? Do you even *like* her?'" She drew a Thespian pause.

Lori swallowed hard. She cringed at the thought of what his response might have been at this point, as he was either being brutally honest with Angela or putting up a defensive barrier and lying through his teeth. Either way, she knew he had nothing to lose by saying something guarded, something less than flattering. She felt her ego blink its blood-shot, watery eyes before shutting them tightly to block out the impending blow.

Angela coughed, as though her throat was lacking moisture from her uninterrupted monologue. "So he paused, Lori, as if he had to *think* about whether or not he liked you, and then he said, '… Y-yeaaaah. I like her.' And then I said, 'But no better or worse than anyone else?' And he paused again and said, 'Y-yeaaaah. I guess you could say that.' What a *jerk*!"

Lori felt her heart dive off its perch and land on her cement-hard stomach, shattering into many pieces and taking pieces of her stomach with it like a suicide bomber. Why did Angela do this? Why did she throw all of these rhetorical questions out, scoop up the ridiculously predictable answers, and then shove them into Lori's face? Was there some kind of ulterior motive behind this Barbara Walters/ academy award-status vulture attack?

"Lori," Angela said, reading into her silence. "I hope this makes you feel better. I mean, how could it not? The guy is a *loser*! All you're guilty of is getting caught up in his *crap*!"

"Uh-huh." Lori said, monotone.

"I told him he'd better not come onto me or to you anymore. I told him that you realized that you made a huge mistake, and that we're more than onto his shallow, one-track, get-a-piece-of-ass-at-all-costs game," she said.

"Thank you."

"The only thing that I'm concerned about," Angela said, taking a deep breath, "is this…"

"What?"

"Sharon Warsaw at the station, who's a good friend of mine, told me that Nick was boasting to her, as well as to the entire station, about your Desiree Jones masquerade."

"He … what?"

Angela made a tsk-tsk noise before saying in a lecturing tone, "The downfall with doing pranks like this, Lori, is making yourself look like some kind of unstable, psycho stalker… I mean I'm sure in time it'll all blow over. But for now, I would just keep a really low profile."

Lori thanked Angela for being such a concerned friend by going to great lengths to get all of this information to her. And then she hung up the phone and contemplated the grossest, messiest form of suicide she could think of.

From: SeriousSchmendrick4428@aol.com
Subject: It makes its own sauce when you add water
To: LoriSolomon6697@yahoo.com
Lori,
Don't worry about being the object of gossip. People can gossip about ME from now till next Tuesday and I wouldn't give a crap. SCREW 'EM! I guarantee you that sending Nick those "Desiree" e-mails gave him a good ego-stroke though. You like that guy, don't you…
I got a message from Jill telling me that she's going to get MARRIED to that androgynous dyke she's been shacked up with for the last year. They're going to have a "commitment ceremony" in Provincetown, Massachusetts this summer. There's no way in HELL

I'm going to miss that! Wonder if she still wants my sperm.

Anyway... I'm laughing too hard to be serious right now. I mean... What should I buy Jill and Gina for a "commitment" present? A fondue pot? Or a double-sided dildo?

WEEEEE!!!

Rutherford

The following day, Lori phoned Angela at her workplace, where she caught her in the middle of an over-the-line feed discussion with Nick. Lori could hear him boasting to Angela over an intercom about his adeptness in pleasing the 'ladies.' She also heard him mention Lori's name, and the fact that she had loved everything he had ever done to her.

"Lori," Angela said to her over the phone. "Nick wants you to vouch for him that he's good 'down there.'"

"Down where?" Lori asked, coolly.

She could hear Nick say, "Tell her to come over here. I'll show her."

Lori wondered if his short-term memory had been completely destroyed by the excessive amounts of heavy-hitting hallucinogens he had taken throughout his life. She suspected that they must have been robust enough and consumed at a high enough frequency to cause such striking brain damage. Brain damage that would cause him to forget that he had sadistically sucked the life force out of another human being only days prior to wanting to mount the same putrefying carcass he helped create.

Who was he?

The weeks passed sluggishly by, and Lori was weary. Her weariness came from sadness. She was exhausted from fighting off feelings that she did not want to have. She was weakened from trying to steer her mind away from the same inane thoughts that served no purpose other than to frustrate her. Yet the upside of her emotional exhaustion was that it made her harmless; it kept her at bay. It was the stainless steel armor that was keeping her palace chaste, unsullied and serene. A slowly blossoming apathy was the sword that was stabbing the beating heart of the raging beast within.

Lori wondered if passion was always fleeting, and if the knowledge of it being fleeting was what drew so much anger out of people. Why was it that the people in Lori's life, including Lori herself, could only feel deeply when provoked? Why were those she thought the least about so solid and stable? Why were the ones she thought the most about uncontrollable and unpredictable? Was passion fueled by mistrust, or the anticipation of resentment? Was it fueled by the angry resentment that follows feelings of hurt or betrayal? She wondered if she could only picture herself clawing and tearing at the flesh of those who had wounded her, biting hard and hungrily into the skin of those who had wronged her, just so she could feel the sweet revenge of momentarily gaining their submission. And she wondered if passion was, in its most heightened form, a kind of sweet revenge.

New Year's Day would soon arrive, and Lori was set on spending it with her two best friends, even though both of them hadn't been in touch with each other for months. Each seemed to have enough to preoccupy them during the time they hadn't spoken for the harsh feelings to subside. Rutherford's nightly cuddling up to frosty cans of Wachusett beer apparently served to tame any residual emotion he may have still harbored toward the situation. Similarly, it seemed that time had washed away a lot of Angela's anger toward Rutherford, especially with fate having dropped "Ted" into her lap, the latest man to aggravate the hell out of her.

"You're an ass, Ted!" Angela had screamed drunkenly into the phone as Rutherford stood in the front doorway of Lori's apartment, tightly clutching his overnight bag.

"Friggin' ass!" She twisted the extension cord around her waist and walked backward through a shuttered door leading into a guest bedroom.

Rutherford hesitantly stepped inside the apartment, watching quietly as Lori swept dust balls away from the radiator in the front hallway.

"You don't have to do that on my account," he said.

"This place is gross. Let me just get some of this crap cleared away."

Rutherford heard a light scratching sound against the entrance behind him, and he turned around to see an exotic-looking girl with a nose piercing and purple-dyed hair leaning her head against a mezuzah nailed into Lori's wooden door frame.

"Hey, Lori!" the girl said.

"Natalie!" Lori dropped her broom and ran over to her former neighbor, whom she had met a month or so earlier, on the day Lori's gray long-haired hamster, resembling at the time a Bubonic Plague-infected rat, had crawled through a crack in the wall and ended up on a living room snack table two stories down. She knew there was only one reason for Natalie to have visited her, uninvited. And it had little to do with auld lang syne, at least in the wholesome sense.

While Angela worked herself up to the point of near regurgitation with her castrating over-the-phone rants, Natalie sat on top of the window seats that lined the bottom of Lori's living room bay window and stared wistfully out at the snow-covered streets. It was there that she waited for Ben, her ex-boyfriend as well as ex-roommate, to appear in the walkway leading to the basement apartment they had recently shared.

"I wonder if he'll bring a girl back," Natalie said. "I miss him so much ..."

Rutherford had quietly moved onto Lori's bed, where he leaned his back against a wall and balanced a cup of orange soda on one leg. He glanced briefly at Angela, whose reddened face was still hurling obscenities into the phone receiver, and then his eyes moved shiftily to Natalie, who was sticking her head under a stiff, brittle window shade.

"Ben is like God," Natalie said suddenly, hopping off the window seat and walking over to Rutherford. "Ben *is* God. He's so beautiful."

Rutherford took a slow, cautious sip of soda, and wiped some off of his re-grown beard with the back of his hand.

"I want him so badly," Natalie groaned, kneeling down on the floor and throwing her upper body over the edge of the bed. "I need him."

Angela suddenly slammed the phone down, stumbled into Lori's bathroom, and shut the door behind her. Lori could vaguely hear her murmur more obscenities over the sound of water gushing from a spigot.

"Oh, God, why did he have to leave me!" Natalie wailed. "I love him more than anyone will ever love him in his whole life!"

Rutherford traced the rim of his glass with his thick, calloused finger. He cleared his throat and softly said, "Natalie?"

"What?" She had started sobbing.

"You've got … a …" He cleared his throat again. *"Problem."*

Natalie blinked hard several times. She started shaking her head violently.

"Just 'cause I love someone, I got a problem?" She stood up and walked back over to the bay window to continue her stakeout.

Angela tugged the bathroom door open. She stomped hard across the floor, and frantically fumbled for a bottle of aspirin in her purse.

An hour or so later, Natalie, who had been sitting frighteningly quiet at the window, gasped. She quickly stood up, backed away from it, and turned to face Rutherford and Lori. Her bare, pierced belly inflated and deflated rapidly from underneath her beaded halter top, and she swept a shaky hand through her long, straw-like hair.

"Oh, my GOD! I don't believe it!" she yelled.

"What?" Lori asked.

"Ben! Ben's back! And he's with someone! He's got a girl with him!" She covered her mouth and raced into the front hallway, her tight leather bell-bottoms flapping wildly as she approached the entrance to her old apartment.

Lori soon heard Natalie knocking hard on Ben's door at the base of the stairs. Lori looked over at Rutherford who had laid himself flat on the bed and had begun to breathe loudly into a pillow. Angela had called her ex-boyfriend again behind a wooden, shuttered door in the adjacent room and was grumbling furiously into the receiver.

"I went on the pill for you!" Natalie's voice spanned the length of the outside stairway leading down to the ground floor apartments. "For you, Ben! I went on the pill! For you!"

Lori heard a high-pitched wail, followed by a thump. She sat frozen, uncertain and disoriented, partly waiting to hear what would happen next, and partly wanting to jump in vigilante-style and right whatever wrongs were no doubt being committed. She finally stood up and walked toward the open front door, when she heard the sound of heavy footsteps bounding up the stairs.

Natalie rushed into the apartment, her once-tame, thick head of hair wild and unkempt, and her eyes misty and smeared with black mascara.

"He threw me like a doll!" she hollered. "Like a little doll! He just picked me up and threw me across the hall!" She pushed past Lori and stumbled into the room where Angela was still mumbling curses with gritted teeth.

"I have to use the phone!" Natalie panted. "I have to call 911!"

"Why?" Angela asked, starting to lower the receiver.

"I'm gonna send that bastard to jail! He just threw me ... across the hall ... like a little doll!"

"Ted, I'm going," Angela hissed. She angrily slammed the phone down and handed it over to Natalie.

"Like a little doll," Natalie repeated. She started to dial the emergency help number.

The police arrived and carted Ben away to spend First Night in jail. Natalie sat in stone cold silence on the wooden storage compartment under the bay window, and stared thoughtfully out at the street.

"You've got to move on," Angela said. She knelt down at Natalie's side and breathed plant-wilting alcohol fumes into her face. "Just like I have to move on."

Natalie continued to stare outside the window, focusing on gleaming icicles dangling from the gabled roof like sleeping albino bats.

"My father was abusive," Angela slurred. "Just like Ted."

Natalie shifted her position on the window seats and tried turning her head away from her, almost as if in an attempt to make her disappear.

"You've got to stop letting the dickheads run and ruin your life," Angela said, her voice getting louder. "You keep inviting the dickheads in, I keep inviting the dickheads in. 'Cause they remind us of all those other dickheads who were there before them. And we think we can change them and we try to change them because we never had the chance to change the other dickheads and by having a new dickhead to change we're being given another chance." She refilled an empty glass with peppermint schnapps.

"Would you stop yelling?" Natalie said. "And ... *spitting* on me?"

"I'm just saying ..." Angela began. She placed a toothpick between her lips, and when she started to try to talk again, it fell out from between her lips and into her filled glass.

"You're driving me crazy," Natalie said, standing abruptly and walking away from her.

Lori had almost fallen asleep on her bed, sitting up against a wall, when she saw Natalie approaching her. She opened her itchy eyes widely and blinked hard to get some moisture flowing into them.

"Are you leaving now?" she asked as Natalie drew closer to her bed. Rutherford had woken up only long enough to remove his face from his own saliva to tell a police officer that he heard and saw nothing during the ordeal. He had fallen back into a deep, restful sleep next to Lori, with an empty carton of milk perched upright between his two thick hands.

"I guess so," Natalie said. "Lori?"

"Yes?"

"Do you think Ben might still be willing to take me back … after tonight?" She paused. "Do you think he might give me another chance?"

Chapter 15

Life is a moderately good play with a badly written third act
Truman Capote (1924-1984)

From: SeriousSchmendrick4428@aol.com
Subject: Vicious muthuh
To: LoriSolomon6697@yahoo.com
So you find me interesting when I'm on mushrooms? When I eat those things and start zoning out on reality, it gets very scary, and I end up rambling on like a god damned lunatic. Hey, screw it. If you want to try it sometime, I'd be happy to get you some samples. Magic mushrooms are seasonal, however. They are usually on the market in the fall and the spring. In all honesty, my bud, I think a good mushroom trip would give you a whole new and exciting perspective on your life. Don't laugh... I'm serious. Those things are like gifts from God that allow us to see the world in a way we never realized before. I can't describe it. It's as if there is a sudden and predictable order to what we normally think of as chaotic human interaction. Everything suddenly makes SENSE, although not to the sober reader of what we're experiencing. To the untrained eye, chaos and unpredictability seem to reign, but if you watch really closely, you experience total order. You wanna do it, or what?
Rutherford

From: LoriSolomon6697@yahoo.com
Subject: Vicious muthuh
To: SeriousSchmendrick4428@aol.com
Uh, no.

Working the mixing board on the weekends at the radio station had long lost its appeal to Lori, and any recording work that came her way had become frustratingly scarce. She was also growing tired of relentlessly recording mock biotechnology reports only to be sent away with a long list of critiques by the fussy station's general manager.

She needed to make it real.

She attended a launch party that was being held on behalf of the station's new programming. She swept through the huge reception hall in search of anyone and everyone who could help her, laughing at jokes she did not understand, touching the arms of those she barely knew, and trying to make eye contact with those who she knew did not care to know her. Breaking through the confines of the mundane was what drove her that night and what kept her moving, and touching, and laughing.

She migrated over to Helga like a clown fish seeking out immunity from a sea anemone in a vast sea of sharks. It was good to see a familiar face among such a diverse and intimidating crowd of people, the face of someone she had learned to know and trust.

"So I'm hearing that I might not be asked to voice anymore of the station's commercials," Lori said, a glass of coke in her shaky hand. "I think they're going to go with a former colleague of the general manager. I feel like I'm getting phased out."

"You are," Helga said.

Lori looked at her, waiting for the support Helga used to give to her when she was feeling nervous or insecure.

"How do you think *I* feel?" Helga said, breaking up the silence. "I'm in-house. Full-time. I'm not a former college intern just dabbling with radio in her free time in between classes. And they've never asked *me* to do *any* of the commercials."

"I don't really understand them," Lori said. She swirled her coke and watched bubbles pop at the surface of a chunk of ice.

"That's why, honey ..." Helga started. Her voice was directed toward Lori, but her eyes moved searchingly around the room. "You have to get *out there* if you're serious about breaking into radio. Market yourself. I keep telling you! Don't just depend on this place!"

"But I have so little time to have to first start hunting around," Lori said. "I'm still in school, for Christ's sake."

"Well..." Helga said, shaking her head. "I don't know what to tell you."

Lori paused, and took a sip of her coke. She was picking up on negativity. Jaded negativity. It used to just be ambivalence.

"Jonathan called me last night," Lori said. "Around eight o'clock."

"Jonathan called you?"

Lori nodded.

"For what?"

"He said they really need biotech coverage for the new business format." Lori took a slow sip of her coke. "I mean, it's not exactly carved in stone, but I suppose if I'm looking for something to keep me tied to the place, this could be it."

"You've been talking about doing reports for those guys forever now," Helga said.

"Jonathan said they'll be considering airing them soon."

Helga nodded, expressionless. "Well, I wish you luck," she said, coldly. "The last time I talked to Jonathan, he referred to me as 'passive-aggressive' and went on to lecture me about all the ways that I could fit in better at the station. I guess I could start by shoving a large stick up my butt." She turned to Burt who had just crept in place beside her. She nudged his arm with the back of her hand, forcing him to turn around and give her some attention. Once he did, she turned her back to Lori.

Lori felt a shiver, an uneasy chill that ran from the backside of her neck down to the small of her back. There was something about the radio environment that seemed to make it easy to make friends, but difficult to keep them. A certain degree of vanity and a certain degree of ego, both fueled by unfathomable, deep-rooted insecurity, were what Lori believed drew her to the business in the first place. There was a good chance that the same was true of Helga. And all the subjectivity and flighty favoritism that incessantly danced around them only fed into the insecurity, and made the hollow emptiness inside of each of them echo more loudly.

Lori spotted Nick in an outer hallway. He was dressed in a gray suit and black tie. She saw Jonathan standing not too far away from him, huddled together with a small group of power black suit and tie figures splintered apart by one or two sparkly evening gowns.

She glanced back at Helga before moving coyly toward Jonathan. Jonathan was the co-host of a morning business and finance show that Helga had run the mixing board for on occasion. He was also a financial advisor whose firm was one floor above the soon-to-be launched business station. It was common knowledge that Jonathan had an interest in eventually buying the station, and that he was already an integral force in planning the design of the station's business format.

"I have a lot of respect for you," he had said to Lori the previous night, with a slight southern drawl. "We need someone who can give the listeners insight into the biopharmaceutical industry. I think with your college background and the fact that you're majoring in science, you can do that for us."

She had gotten off the phone with him, dizzy with glee at the prospect of there existing an alternative to a future consisting of transference of clear liquids from one polystyrene tube to another in a gray metal rack on a bench top under long rectangular fluorescent ceiling lights in a room that often smelled of gas or sulfur.

She continued walking toward Jonathan, stopping short of the group of elegance and supremacy that clustered before her. She lightly tapped on his shoulder. He turned around to face her, looking pleasantly surprised to see her. She smiled and leaned toward him and kissed his cheek. His look of pleasant surprise quickly changed over to simply a look of surprise. Lori blushed and stepped back, feeling awkward about what she had just done.

"How are you, Jonathan?" she asked. She hung her head and bashfully looked down at her feet. "I just wanted to tell you how excited I am about the possibility of doing biotechnology updates for the station."

"I can *see* how excited you are!" he said with his trademark drawl. "It's something the station needs, and we're happy to have you on board to do it."

"Thanks," she said. "So it's official? I'm really doing this?"

"So far as I can tell you are," he said. "We'll get you together with the program director sometime in the next couple of weeks, and you guys can work out the details."

"Thanks again," Lori said. "So how soon now before the station's yours?"

"Soon, hopefully," Jonathan said. "I've got some plans. A few things are in the fire."

Lori smiled and shook his hand. She pivoted around in her half-heels, and found herself facing Nick.

She slowly approached him.

"Hello, Lori," he said stiffly. He moved only the lower half of his body to face her, while keeping his head and neck in the same awkward position they had originally been in. It was obvious that formal attire made him skittish.

"So, are you and I O.K. with each other?" she asked, nervously.

"Yeah. Why wouldn't we be?"

"I don't know."

"We're fine," he said. He glanced around the room. "You know, Mona and I broke up. Couple of months ago."

"Angela had told me when it happened."

"Yeah. She decided that she needed space," he said.

Lori looked up at him, searching his face for signs of regret, or sadness. But his icy blue eyes and taut lips looked the same as they always had. Immune. Impervious.

"So where's … Paul?" he asked, interrupting her. He looked thoughtfully around at crowds of people huddled together in the adjacent ballroom.

"Paul?"

"Yeah. How come I've never met this guy? You still with him?"

Lori shrugged, and decided not to answer his question directly. *So you think I'm still seeing Paul,* she thought. *Maybe it's best that I remain just as much of a mystery to you as you've been to me since the day I met you, so we can finally have an even playing field.*

"Ah," he said, obviously attempting to answer his own question despite her silence. "So ... can I be of any ... assistance to you this evening?"

"No," she said. She could feel his eyes on her, even if for only a second before he felt the need to return them to the strangers in the ballroom. Despite his façade, she could still feel his masked loneliness; she could still feel his stifled hurt. Mona was gone, and it was obvious that Mona was very near to being gone when Lori had last seen him. But although it helped her to understand, it didn't take away her own masked loneliness and stifled hurt.

"I do want to do this, though," she said. She stretched her arms out toward him and drew him tightly to herself, wanting at that moment to squeeze all of the bad feelings away, like pinching a pus-filled blemish tightly between one's thumb and forefinger. His hands were lightly perched on her waist, his back still hard and erect. She pulled away from him slowly, and kept her eyes averted and pointed toward the floor. She started moving through the crowds of people away from him.

From: SeriousSchmendrick4428@aol.com
Subject: closure hugs
To: LoriSolomon6697@yahoo.com

Jesus, Lori, you've had nothing but "closure" with that loser for months now. "Closure" hugs, "closure" talks, "closure" this and "closure" that. Closure my ass. You are so hot for that guy it's hilarious to hear you deny it so much. If you weren't, you'd be ignoring him and avoiding him, but instead you're giving him warm huggies. That wasn't exactly the SMARTEST move you could have made if you truly wanted him to go away, you think? You may as well have whispered, "take me," in his ear, because I guarantee you that's the message he got.

Oh, well, I've got my own problems, too. I'm on my way to Kansas City in a few hours. I'm leaving there next Friday, so I can imagine Thursday will be the big "fight" day. Screw it. I just can't wait to get laid.

Rutherford

The days passed lazily by, and Lori was just beginning to feel like her mildly, as opposed to highly, neurotic self once again. It was still difficult for her to envision visiting the radio station, knowing that it was possible that she would see Nick, and knowing there was a chance he would treat her like a large, fetid turd. Yet she felt her strength returning, and also felt the vast bulk of the stinging hurt starting to drift away. She was growing weary of dealing with the recurring, pointless anguish, and there was a good chance that her very fatigue would end up being the best friend she could ever hope to have.

Angela called her one evening in the middle of a tuna and corn chip feast.

"Guess who called me?" she asked.

A small chunk of albacore got caught somewhere between Lori's tonsils and her windpipe. She started to cough and gag.

"Are you all right?" Angela yelled into the phone.

"A-hah!" Lori gasped. She continued coughing for a few more seconds and swallowed hard to push the dry, sticky fish all the way down her throat. "Went down the wrong way," she said in a hoarse whisper.

"Well, I'll continue when I know you're all right," she said.

"I'm all right. Just tell me. Was it Nick?"

"He left a message on my answering machine at home, just to 'say hi' and to 'see how I was.' I didn't get back to him. And I'm not planning to," she said.

"I can picture how he sounded on your machine," Lori said, making her voice high pitched and nasal, and putting on her thickest New England accent. "Yeeaah, so Angela... This is Nick. Yeeaah, so... aftah I kicked my retahdid girlfriend's *ass* outta my dad's basement, I realized that I was missin' the aaah... convahsation you and me used to have. Yeah, so I'm in need of some... *convahsation*. Would you be interested in... aaah... *conversing* with me sometime, Angela?"

"I just hope he doesn't call me again."

"Whatever," Lori said, adding a spoonful of mayonnaise to the tuna. "I'm getting so tired of trying to figure him out. Look, just tell him you're a full-blown lesbian, you and I are lesbian lovers."

"You mean tell him the truth."

Lori was feeling particularly staunch as she walked into the radio station early one evening to work on a piece that was to air that weekend. Nick was sitting quietly at his desk when she breezed past him toward the production studio. He paused only to give her a gentle greeting before turning his attention back to his work.

"Hi," she said softly, picking up her pace. She closed the heavy wooden door behind her, positioned herself in front of the editing equipment and microphone, and began shuffling the papers of script she had brought in with her. She heard a light rapping sound. She looked up and saw Nick's face in a little transom window in the door.

"Hey, I got something for you," he said. He walked inside the room with a sheet of paper in his hand. "A spot for Joe's show this Saturday."

"Thank you." She stood up and pulled it gently from his hands.

"Do you want me to help you?" he asked.

"No. I can do it myself."

"Why?" he asked.

"Because I feel self-conscious reading in front of someone else."

He diverted his glance toward the screen of a nearby computer. He smiled and said, "But I've seen you naked."

She felt a surge of adrenaline strike the pit of her stomach and make it lurch. "I heard you called Angela," she said.

He laughed. "She and I just flirt and kid around. We have fun." He grabbed the chair Lori had been sitting on and began to prepare the production equipment for the read. He looked up at her. "I could see down your shirt before."

Lori glanced down at the V-necked polo shirt she was wearing, and saw only the fabric lining her collar tight against her clavicle.

"I can touch you," he said. He pointed his finger at her chest.

"No, you can't."

"Why not?"

"Because I'm over all that," she said. She was surprised at what was coming out from between her lips, as it bore no resemblance to anything that was going on in her head or her heart.

"Okay," he said, briskly. He looked away from her and rose to leave.

"Could you explain something?" Her mouth was moving before she knew what was to come out of it.

"Sure, what?" he said.

"Why were you so nasty to me the last time we were together? When I drove you to the train station that one night?"

"What do you mean?" He looked puzzled.

"When I asked you to tell me something about yourself, you told me that I had no reason to know anything about you," she said, blinking hard. The memory was flashing at her full force.

"I didn't say it like *that*!" he shouted, backing away toward the door. He smiled nervously at her.

"That's what I heard."

"That's not what I said." He continued to look at her for a few seconds, grinning stupidly. He walked out of the room.

Lori completed the commercial read, and then walked over to his desk and asked him to load it into the station's system for her. He marched into the production studio, his head bowed. He went through the motions very fast. He did not look at her or even face her. He just finished, and headed toward the door.

"Bye!" Lori called out to him.

He said nothing and disappeared around the corner.

From: SeriousSchmendrick4428@aol.com
Subject: Numb nuts
To: LoriSolomon6697@yahoo.com

Jehovah's Witnesses approached me today. They're lovely people, well meaning and friendly, and they're CRAZY! I just don't understand these weirdo Christian sects like the JW's and the 7th Day Adventists and the Mormons... not to mention the Irish Republican Army, which I'm technically a member of. TECHNICALLY. I've never been to church in my whole friggin' life, so how is it that I'm considered an Irish Catholic just because my ancestors were? I wouldn't know a Holy Rosary from a

Snicker's Bar. And why is it that corned beef is so prominent on St. Patrick's Day? I usually associate corned beef with the infamous Reuben sandwich, which is a Jewish New York Deli creation. I just don't get it. Rutherford (a.k.a. Crafty Barnardo)

Lori's eyes opened at three o'clock in the morning. She lay flat on her back, motionless, staring up at some ceiling cracks, and began to recall every single person or non-person in her life that had ever hurt or wronged her over the years. Merciless hectors that had exploited her shyness as a child, heartless cretins that had ridiculed her for not being beautiful, past love-interests who had turned their backs on her for not being lovable enough, family that had criticized, acquaintances that had degraded, strangers that had insulted, dogs that had bitten. It gravely concerned her how easy it was for her mind to pluck from the vast reservoir of life experiences such blatant negativity, and how pristinely preserved the bad memories were after all of the time that had passed.

She wasn't sure what had triggered it, if it were a dream or a nightmare or a peppery food she had eaten before she climbed into bed for the night. All she knew was that it was all there, perched and ready in its typically dormant state to leap out at her unexpectedly and make her feel- at least for the moment- that life can be one pain-in-the-ass.

Lori flung the bed covers off and restlessly folded her pillow over underneath her head and shoulders so that she was partly sitting up. Her brain was pulsating rapidly beneath her skull, and her body was filled with pent-up libido energy in dire need of an outlet that was nowhere to be found. She wondered if bread would still rise if she injected the contents of an old tube of

Monistat 7 into a mound of freshly prepared dough. She wondered if the rumors were true that she heard as a child, that she would turn into a black hole if she tried to simultaneously belch, sneeze, and hiccup. She wondered how big of an object in her apartment she was capable of picking up with her toes. She wondered if there would be a change in her stool color if she ate nothing but vegetables for a week, then nothing but beef for a week.

She staggered over to her computer, hoping to lose her self-indulgent thoughts somewhere in the chaotic whirlwind of someone else's universe. She felt effortless joy when her eyes fell on the number "2" sitting temptingly in her e-mail "inbox." She decided to first read a message she had received from Pista Bakfark, who was responding to an e-mail she had sent him the previous week. It was obvious from his steady decline in the ability to write intelligible English sentences that he was speaking only Uralic in his native country.

He Lori,
Did I just speak out that you are simply and truly the sweetest thing on the surface of that planet. I was just reading again what you were writing some days ago, in fact, I had to read it again, and once you'll also read it again you simply know why I truly call you the sweetest thing. I kiss the sweat from all over your naked body (esp. from your inner thighs where it is even sweeter).
I kiss your boobies! (I mean both of them!)
Just missing to go on your nerves. Just missing to expose myself to you. Just missing you, but NOT missing that stupid lab for a single second.
I was just phantasizing about our 'sordid past', was just finding myself getting totally aroused. I mean squezing

and striking myself, just getting offffffffffffff, oooohhh Jezzzzzzzz, I mean …
Love ya,
P.B.

Dear Pista,
Do you know what "striking" means? You said that you were punching yourself. Did you mean, "stroking?" Also, "fantasizing" is spelled with an "f," and "squeezing" is spelled with two "es."
Lori

She moved quickly to a message from Rutherford. She hoped that his innate cynicism and sarcasm would tap into her uneasy state of mind and bring her some much needed relief.

From: SeriousSchmendrick4428@aol.com
Subject: ectopic pregnancy gone badly
To: LoriSolomon6697@yahoo.com
God dammit! I was just writing you a message and friggin' AOL logged me off for "inactivity." Did you get it? I can't BELIEVE how much AOL SUCKS!!!!! WHY do they do that!?
I'm kind of worked up right now, baby. A little while ago I almost got into a FIGHT with some idiot in a parking lot near here. To make a long story short, I was about to make a turn in the lot, and this guy was coming in the opposite direction and stopped in front of me rather than driving by. I waved with my hand as if to say "go ahead" or "you first" or whatever, and this little punk-ass drove past me and hung his head out the window and said "Use your directional, schmuck!" I couldn't believe it! He went by me and I did a U-turn and pulled up to his truck after he parked, and I very calmly said "Dude, don't you think it's a little stupid to talk to people that

way?" This clown looked like he weighed about 130 pounds, and he says "Whatchya gonna do about it!" Oh my God! I swear, I was so mad after that I almost jumped out of my car to beat that jerk within an inch of his life, but I got hold of my testosterone and I just shook my head and said, "You ain't even worth it," and I left. Why? WHY do sawed-off little punks like that talk like friggin tough guys to someone MY size? I swear, in my life, I've been challenged to fight by maybe five or six different guys, and they're ALWAYS guys that are about HALF as big as me!

Oh well, I think I did the right thing by walking away. I don't want to have to answer my e-mails from a prison computer.

Rutherford

From: LoriSolomon6697@yahoo.com
Subject: Re:
To: SeriousSchmendrick4428@aol.com

You did the right thing. You fought fire with fire. Hauled off some obscenities in return for the obscenities he hauled off on you. Feel sorry for the jerk. He obviously had a bug up his butt over SOMETHING. What sucks is that people whose lives suck make things difficult for the rest of us.

Lori

She happily sent her message off to Rutherford and was just about to log off, when her eyes fell on a message that must have just been sent to her from Angela. It was twenty minutes after three in the morning. What was she doing awake?

From: AngelontheAirwaves3254@hotmail.com
Subject: Re:
To: LoriSolomon6697@yahoo.com

Hello my Lovely Lesbian Lover,

Sorry I couldn't see you last night; I was tired and depressed all weekend. Don't really know why. I think I'm lonely and horny... Haven't heard anything from Ted ... I did hear from Stanley, my otherwise "unavailable" friend. But it was just a joke that he sent to all his e-mail buddies. I didn't respond. I'm done with him. I know he's more miserable than ever in his relationship. Why won't he leave her for me????? Now that is someone I am absolutely HOT for in every possible way. Life is not fair, Lori. Why can't I find a guy whom I am attracted to and LIKE at the same time????? It's always either one or the other!!!

Love,

Your LL/SF

From: LoriSolomon6697@yahoo.com
Subject: Re:
To: AngelontheAirwaves3254@hotmail.com

I don't know why life has to suck so badly. What I do know is, with Stanley, you must ask yourself ONCE AGAIN the same question I keep asking myself: Why are you time and time again attracted to these insurmountable, self-defeatist challenges? What about that nice guy Ron who you went out on some dates with a while back? I mean, what was wrong with him? He was single, outgoing ... Or what about Jerry? The one I introduced you to? What ever happened there? He didn't seem so bad to me. It seems like we both push the promising ones away, and gravitate toward the ones that are nothing but trouble.

Anyway, we've got to talk. There's a lot more I'd like to say on this subject!!

Your L.L./S.F.,

Lori

Lori sent the message to Angela with the intent of turning off the computer and trying to fall back to sleep, when her eyes fell on a new message from Rutherford. Insomnia seemed to be running rampant that night.

From: SeriousSchmendrick4428@aol.com
Subject: It's slinky ... It's slinky ...
To: LoriSolomon6697@yahoo.com
You ain't kidding about how people with miserable lives make it tough on the rest of us. Jesus, all I wanted to do was stop at a sub-shop and pick up a pizza and go on my merry way, and because of that knucklehead I almost got into a friggin fistfight. Can you imagine? I'd have either been ARRESTED for beating the guy senseless, OR he'd have pulled out a gun and shot my ass. Where's the LOVE, god dammit!
I'm getting a crush on this chick that works at Dipstick Donuts, by the way. I stop in there every night and get a donut and chocolate milk for the mentally retarded guy I'm taking care of, and this girl is always so bubbly and friendly and jiggly-wiggly. Tonight she was asking me about what I do for a living, and I gave her a quick run-down. She said something like, "Aw, that's nice, you must have a big heart to work with disabled people." I felt like saying, "My heart ain't the ONLY thing I've got that's big, baby," but I held my tongue. God, I'm a pervert. That chick is probably about sixteen years old.
Well, I'm outta here. As always, I'll speak with thee expediently and with much Godspeed.
P.S. OY!
Rutherford

Lori switched her computer off and lay down in her bed again. She finally fell asleep. The sound of her ringing phone awakened her the following morning.
"Hello?"

Rutherford's voice sounded strained to Lori on the other end of the phone line. "I know this is kinda short notice, but can you come for a visit this weekend?"

"I read all your e-mails last night. To what do I owe all this sudden attention?"

"I'm needy." He laughed. "No, seriously, can you come up here for a visit?"

"Uh... Maybe. I don't know. I'm kind of tired," she said, feeling the weight even of just the receiver in her hand. "I don't know if I'll have enough energy to drive all the way into New Hampshire. As you well know, I had a lousy night's sleep. So did you, apparently."

"Look," he said. "Without getting into detail here, I'd just appreciate the company."

There was something about being needed and depended upon that gave Lori a strong sense of warmth, like sitting in front of an open, roaring fire, cloaked in a soft comforter. She felt the same rush of fulfillment then as she had months earlier, when Rutherford had phoned her at four in the morning to seek advice about an inebriated friend of his who had urinated into the vegetable compartment of his refrigerator. Perhaps the strange, befuddled high she would get was due to knowing deep down inside how unstable of a character that she, herself, was, and yet having people in turmoil actually leaning on *her* for strength.

That night, she drove to see Rutherford. Grinning, saliva-dripping dust bunnies swirled around her feet when she stepped inside his apartment. She neared a grease-splattered ping-pong table covered with stale cake and cookie crumbs and looked for a chair to sit in.

"Make yourself at home," Rutherford said. He pointed at the ping-pong table.

"Didn't you used to have a real kitchen table here?" she asked.

"Yeah. Termites," he said. "Can I get you something?" he asked.

"Oh, no.... No," Lori said. She knew that he was knee-deep in a phase in which he was experimenting with various exotic foods that included obscure crustaceans and candy-coated insects. Obviously bored with cheese, he had been talking about getting Lori to try a strawberry syrup-dipped grasshopper, or a scorpion frozen motionless in the center of a square butterscotch flavored lollypop.

He reached his hand into a metal cooking pot of white and green mushrooms. "I want to be lowered into a shark cage." He carried a plate of growth over to the ping-pong table and sat across from her. "Saw these guys doing it on T.V. Looks pretty cool."

"You wouldn't be scared?" Lori asked.

"Only maybe when it comes to paying the bill. Whoo!" He shoved some mushrooms into his mouth. He shifted in his chair and pushed his emptied plate to one side of the ping-pong table.

"Hey, I'm thinking about becoming a voo-doo priest. What do you think about that?"

Lori smiled. "I think that one of the things we both have in common is a constant need for stimulation and change. Or else we get bored."

"True …" he said, smacking his lips. He stood up and walked over to the pot of mushrooms sitting on a stove burner. "You absolutely sure I can't get you anything?"

"Yes," she said. "I'm really not hungry. But thanks."

He quietly stirred the mushrooms, flipping them with a spatula over and over until Lori believed he was only doing it to keep himself busy. He added a pinch of some kind of seasoning, before wiping his hands on his fatigues.

"Things suck," he said. "And things just keep sucking. Things in my life increase in suckiness every day by a factor of ten, at least. Life is a suppository in the rectum of the universe."

"Life just keeps going on and on and on, doesn't it?" Lori said.

"Things suck. But right now, whatever. Don't care. Screw it," he said.

"So what sucks, exactly?" she asked.

"What doesn't?" He continued flipping mushrooms over and over with the spatula. "Got to go in for surgery on my back."

"Really? That's... That's right," she said. "You mentioned you were in pain the last time I talked to you."

"Yeah. Spinal surgery. They're going to check to see if I have one." He started laughing loudly, and then put on a fake Indian accent. "Yah, Mistuh Jones... We haf gone in and looked, and haf discovuhed dat you haf no spine! You wimpy bastaaad!"

They segued into discussing the general futility of life as both of them saw it. How often Rutherford couldn't help but venture off into such extremist thrill-seeking behavior that he found himself tinkering on the edge of self-destruction, all for the purpose of warding off stagnation. Lori was just beginning to get heated up, clawing at what she perceived to be a whisper of justification for her own recurring adventurism, when the tides of the conversation shifted toward Rutherford's unyielding hopelessness and regret. Regret over lost loves, lost career pursuits, a perceived lost life. Lori had tried many times to bring Rutherford's mind to the forefront of the present, even pushed it on occasion and tried to get him to contemplate a future for himself. He was still so young, yet he talked like he was an old man. He insisted on lamenting over that which was gone, that which could do nothing but immobilize him like an institutional straight jacket.

"So are you O.K.?" Lori asked.

"Me? Yeah…"

"Are you sure?" Lori asked.

"Yeah," he said, chuckling. "I mean ... life just… sucks, you know? I've seen so much… so much and it all just… sucks."

"I know," she said.

"People out there… just going through the motions. Not giving a crap about anyone other than themselves, not really giving a crap about anything, you know? People just suck."

"I know," she said.

"There's no such thing as morals anymore. People are jerks, they know they're jerks, and they just don't care that they're jerks. They do things just because they can. Not because they should. Society has never been as selfish, corrupt, and depraved as it is now."

"Yes."

"And it's the selfishness, the corruption, the depravity that is tearing down any sense of union or structure that society may have once had," he said. "We're individuals struggling for more and more individuality, constantly justifying our selfish, corrupt, depraved crap, rationalizing that it's simply our right as individuals to be this way."

"Yeah."

"Lord, I'm good with words," he said. "Hey, guess what?"

"What?"

I have a new… suspicious… *mole*." He laughed.

"Have you had it checked?" she asked.

"Nah," he said, continuing to laugh. "Screw it."

"You should get it looked at."

"You know, there's something I need to let you know."

"What's that?" she asked.

He dug underneath the mushrooms with the spatula and lifted a group of them high in the air. Letting them fall erratically from a lofty height back into the pot, he said, "I'm attracted to you."

Lori felt her face grow warm.

He looked at her then, while continuing to stir the pot.

She shifted her eyes toward the table and focused on a box of cheese danishes. She wondered if there were any pastries still inside of it, and if they were moldy or stale. She thought about the Dipstick Donuts girl. She thought about Babette. She thought about Angela. She thought about what it's like to be alone.

"You got pretty quiet," Rutherford said, laughing. He reached over his head and pulled a plastic bowl out of a cupboard. He began filling it up with seasoned mushrooms.

"Well …" Lori started. She paused for a moment to collect her thoughts. "I think … that you're just ready to be with someone."

"Y…eah …" he said. He nodded and continued to toss mushrooms from the pot into the plastic bowl.

"It's been a long time for you, and you're just feeling lonely," she said. "And I think we're too good of friends to let a moment like this ruin what we've had for so many years. Don't you think?"

Rutherford covered the bowl with plastic wrap and set it in the refrigerator. "Hey, would you like to … see this book that I just got?"

They moved to his cluttered living room where he pulled out some writing guides that he had picked up at a yard sale. They carried on with their evening as though nothing had happened. Yet something *had* happened. It was something that she feared. And it was also something that she sort of, kind of, craved. It was something that she sort of, kind of, craved *because* it was something that she feared.

Rutherford knew this. He could tell from the gleam she had in her eyes when she talked about Nick. He could tell from the sparkle that was still in her eyes when she berated herself for letting it happen. Rutherford knew that Lori was attracted to the randomness of peril. He also knew that he, himself, was wrought with danger and uncertainty, the very qualities that Lori found irresistible. He knew all he needed to know, and it was just enough for him to bathe Lori in her own juices, and stir her like a steaming pot of his sautéed mushrooms.

From: AngelontheAirwaves3254@hotmail.com
Subject: Re:
To: LoriSolomon6697@yahoo.com
Lori, I want to follow up on something you wrote to me recently that kinda disturbed me. Don't worry. This is not a criticism. I just really want to set the record straight with you about certain guys in my past that I rejected. You brought up Ron and Jerry the other night, and it really threw me for a loop. Lori, I really, REALLY need you to understand that you are WAY off base here, and this is truly NOT my being in denial about anything. The guys I have rejected- like Ron and Jerry- were SO FAR beneath my standards in so many ways that I could not, SIMPLY COULD NOT, bring myself to settle for them. Not only did they all mentally/emotionally repulse me, but they physically repulsed me as well. You apparently never noticed how completely rank and nasty Ron was. Well, my friends at work met him once, and they were like, "Angela, for God's sake you can do better than THAT. That guy is

gross." My friend Jack Wiener actually welled up a bit when he asked me why I felt I had to "settle" for guys like that. And when I described his disgusting living conditions, both Jack and my other pal at work, Mark Pigeon, said they couldn't even listen. Lori, the guy was THE BOTTOM OF THE BARREL. He stank. His breath smelled like I don't know what. He smoked cigarettes AND pot, and the list goes on and on. And further, he ADMITTED to me that he had "intimacy issues" and had never been in a long-term relationship. You REALLY think I should have continued to see this guy? I could not give Jerry a chance because again, I just would not allow myself to sink that low. He didn't seem clean, his teeth were awful (and he had bad breath), he was disheveled and way overweight. And he was ALL about himself the night I met him, never ONCE asking me a bloody question about ME. I am sorry, but at least the guys I find myself genuinely wanting to be with have been light years ahead of the aforementioned two- physically, emotionally, and mentally.

I think one reason people like Ron and Jerry don't seem as "nasty" to you as they do to me is because, as you've admitted, you kind of have a hippy side to you. And I definitely do not. Like, you wore jeans with huge holes in them for a while, and that's just something I would never do. And neither would I want to date a guy who wore such clothes. Of course, I have no problem with YOU wearing torn jeans or anything else- because you are not a potential love interest. And besides, you are a basically clean person who bathes regularly and brushes her teeth! You take CARE of yourself, and always look attractive and appealing. Ron and Jerry do not. I just hope you understand, and don't think me shallow for feeling as I do. I also happen to think the outer is a reflection of the inner, and if the outer is a mess, you can make a pretty good guess that the inner

is a mess as well. When people are happy with themselves, it usually shows in their appearance.
Gotta go do the TRAFFIC now.
Love ya!

Chapter 16

Reality is merely an illusion, albeit a very persistent one
Albert Einstein (1879-1955)

The last slice of pizza lay untouched in the cardboard box it came in, the cheese on its surface having turned into a rough, lukewarm rubbery sheet. Three empty coke cans surrounded it on Lori's coffee table, partly shadowed by an imposing half empty bottle of Madeira wine Lori had swiped from her uncle's house. Lori was leaning lazily against the arm of her couch, while Marta sat cross-legged on the hardwood floor.

"It's star 82 to block our number, or theirs?" Marta asked, lifting the phone receiver to her jaw and trying to untangle the attached cord.

"No," Lori said. "Star 67 blocks our number from being seen by someone else. Star 69 lets you call someone back if they call you and hang up without saying anything. And star 82 counter blocks a block that prevents unregistered calls, like from phone solicitors, from getting through."

"It's a strange world we're living in, is it not?" Marta asked.

Lori shrugged and nodded. "I was wearing a retainer the last time I did something like this."

"Yes? And?" Marta said, raising her palms toward the ceiling. "Who cares? Who's going to know?"

Lori shrugged.

"Since when should fun be reserved only for children?" Marta asked, flipping her short dark wisps of hair out from underneath her shirt collar. "Let's see. Let me find the Swiss guy's number for you." She lowered the phone to her lap and pulled a folded white sheet of notebook paper out of her purse. "Still haven't gotten myself a proper address book," she said, laughing.

"You'd think something like that would be important for a European attending college in the United States to have, eh?" She took a sip of wine and began dialing the digits of her former beau. She handed the phone to Lori.

"Please leave a message and a phone number, and I'll get back to you as soon as possible," a male voice announced with a mild accent.

Lori cleared her throat. "Is this … Dick's Eatery?" Her voice was rich and sultry. She tried to suppress her drunken laughter as she went through the script in the same exaggeratedly theatrical way she would have if it were going on air as a commercial. When she finished, she handed the phone to Marta.

"O.K. Who's next?"

Lori thumbed through her little black address book for Nick's number. She had to copy it from a laminated list of personnel at the radio station, since she had destroyed any numbers that he had personally given to her months ago.

Marta pressed star 67, followed by his number, and waited. Her forehead creased and she mouthed, "answering machine," to Lori.

"Hi," she said in her sweet, soft Italian voice. "I'm … I'm not sure if this is the right number, or not. But … I was looking for Dick's Eatery. I was wondering if you had anything for my friend and me to *eat*."

Lori pulled a pillow close to her and squeezed a corner of it.

"You know," Marta continued. "Bite, suck, chew … *swallow*. Something … soft. Well, actually," she said, chuckling. "*Hard* is what we're really looking for. A … Popsicle … or … a hot dog …"

She covered the receiver and let out a silent laugh. "Something creamy and rich. Or maybe … meaty. Hot and tasty. I'll get back to you, because we're really, *really* hungry."

It was just past eleven at night when Marta rose to leave. She was going to see a boy named "Matteo," whom she had met several months earlier through the Internet. Marta and Matteo saw each other infrequently in person, yet flirted on an almost daily basis through an "instant messenger" service.

"So I asked him why he never returns my calls when I leave him messages on his answering machine," Marta said. "And he tells me he's just not a 'phone person.'" She swung the thin black strap of her purse over her tiny shoulder. "He spends every waking hour on the Internet," she said. "I can only communicate with him if it's in the form of writing. I tell you, it's not normal."

After Marta left, Lori cleared away some pizza crumbs and dishes and lay down on her couch. She pointed her remote control at her television, and began flipping from one channel to the next in rapid succession. Nothing interested her. Her eyelids started to droop, and she closed them. The blare of the television was keeping her awake. She fumbled in vein for the remote control, and surrendering, recoiled under an afghan and tried to block out the noise.

The phone rang. It was still on the floor near the coffee table where Marta had been sitting. Lori lifted her head out from under the afghan and stared at it. Keeping the afghan wrapped around her shoulders, she bent down to pick it up.

"Hello?"

"Hello. Is Lori there?"

"Oh, God ..."

"So you rang?" Nick said.

"It was my friend. We were drunk."

"Is she cute?" he asked.

"Yes," Lori said. "We used star 67. Did my number come up on your end?"

"No," he said. "I just knew it was you."

She nodded.

"So ... what are you wearing?" he asked.

Lori smiled, trying to push her lethargy away just enough to be conscious of the moment. "Sweats," she said. "And a white tee-shirt."

"Bra?"

"Yes," she said. "What about you?"

"I'm wearing my boxers."

"The blue ones?" she asked.

"Yes," he said softly. "The blue ones."

"I remember those."

"Picture me there with you," he said. "I come up behind you.... I start kissing your neck ... your ear ..."

He went on to talk dirty to her, very dirty, and tried to get her to envision the two of them together ... being dirty, *very* dirty. She stayed on the phone with him, lying languidly in the middle of the living room's hardwood floor and staring directly into a light fixture on the ceiling. She felt as though she were dreaming, yet was in too deep to wake herself out of it. She told him that the wine and pizza had made her very tired, too tired to continue what he was trying to start. Yet she remained on the phone.

"... your pink passion pit," he said.

"Pink *passion pit*?" she repeated, laughing loudly.

He ignored her and continued. "My hand is on your ..."

She lay there with one arm outstretched, and the receiver wedged in between her chin and shoulder. She emancipated it only after a considerable amount of time passed, when a torrent of energy dissipated and left her feeling listless and weak.

It was then that she realized that whatever was going on inside her was not simple childishness, or anything that she was capable of simply tying up in an unassuming carton and shoving far under her bed amidst clutter and balls of dust. It was something very serious, very insidious, and very undeniably real.

From: SeriousSchmendrick4428@aol.com
Subject: self-pleasure is the best pleasure
To: LoriSolomon6697@yahoo.com
I'm glad you mentioned your attempts to prank call me last night. My parents have been HERE very frequently lately, especially on Friday and Saturday and Sundayses. In a word, if you call here looking to prank me on the wrong night, the joke might be on YOU. My parents are actually very laid-back and wouldn't yell at you or anything (in fact, my father might even LIKE to answer the phone late at night and hear a female voice saying she was looking for something long and hard and creamy). But just be warned. It might not be ME that picks up the phone.
My vacation with Babette went differently than I'd expected. We didn't really have any "fights" at all. However, I must say, after the "honeymoon" period during the first five days, I was suddenly SEIZED with the torment of wanting to get the HELL outta there. The last two days in Kansas City ALL I could think about was how much I wanted to go the hell home, you know? That girl was irritating the CRAP out of me. I know it sounds bizarre and egomaniacal, but the only reason I can't bring myself to completely break it off with her is because I feel so BAD for her. She's obviously completely attached to my stupid ass, and I just don't want to hurt her feelings, god dammit. The fact that we

live so far away from each other is the ONLY reason I haven't told her to get lost by now. If I had to be around her every day, there's no way in hell I could stand it. The funny thing is... the more I blow her off and act like a complete jerk, the more she seems to get attached to me! Jesus...

Oh well. Work SUCKS! I HATE it! If you never worked with retarded people, you just wouldn't understand.

Rutherford

P....S.... Give the Nick crap a REST! You're like a freakin' Jr High School girl prank-calling her dream-boy for Christ's sake! If you really aren't obsessing over that blathering dickhead, then WHY do you keep interacting with him? Why?

The days of the week were beginning to pass by at a decent enough pace. Lori went to her classes in the mornings, studied at home in the afternoons. She paused from her routine only to occasionally peer into her e-mail and open friends' messages left in her "inbox." Nick Warren had sent her nothing new, yet this did not concern her- at least initially. His puzzling, and at the same time predictable, absence had no adverse effect on her ego or her psyche until around mid-week, when she found herself thinking about how their phone conversation had made her feel that steamy, searing night as she lay euphoric on the dusty hardwood floor of her living room.

From: Lori Solomon6697@yahoo.com
so ... i'm fine for MONTHS, then you get my motor running again
what exactly are we to each other?

From: NickWarren557@hotmail.com
playmates

Playmates. The word suggested innocence. Fun and freedom. Thanks to Nick, there was a whole magical underworld of possibilities that Lori would know nothing about had she not considered straying somewhat from the so-called norm. And the wonder of this virtually uncharted universe would be enough to carry her, if she had the discipline to take only small tastes of it from time to time. If she could sneak tiny bites that were little more than pleasing to her palate, then she believed that she could enjoy this world. Yet Lori knew that she could easily indulge too much, engulf too fast. When teased with only a morsel, Lori tended to want the entire dish. The contingency of this world, if Lori wanted it to last, was restraint. After all, it was fleeting passion. Recurring passion, but fleeting passion all the same. To enjoy it as it were, she would always have to feel a certain degree of hunger. And at times, perhaps even starvation.

From: Lori Solomon6697@yahoo.com
then play with me

From: NickWarren557@hotmail.com
SAY THE WORD AND I WILL

The exchanges continued for several days more. Lori sent messages out, and Nick responded only seconds after receiving them. Unable to resist the instant gratification of opening these gates to sex-splashed adventure, Lori periodically slipped out from underneath her papers and textbooks to check for e-mail messages on her computer. The longer it continued, the more she wondered if Nick's sense of equilibrium and control were being compromised to nearly the same extent as her own.

Her heart would sloppily fold upon itself whenever she would see no immediate response after sending him a message. Part of his game seemed to be keeping her guessing, by suddenly and inexplicably not responding to her.

From: Lori Solomon6697@yahoo.com
so are we done playing? or do you want to continue?

She held her breath as she exited her e-mail, and then she began busying herself with a magazine that she lifted from her desk. Helplessly, she logged back into her account and let out a long, relieved exhale as her eyes fell on the number "1" sitting in her inbox. The only thing that could kill the ecstasy of the moment would be if the number "1" corresponded to one of her uncle Hyman's many forwarded Jewish jokes or blanket political e-mails.

From: NickWarren557@hotmail.com
what shall we do next? the real thang?

From: Lori Solomon6697@yahoo.com
is that what you want?

From: NickWarren557@hotmail.com
yeah

Lori sighed heavily and rested her forehead against the computer screen. She had been hurt before. Why should she be spared now?

From: Lori Solomon6697@yahoo.com
i liked that phone conversation we had a week ago

From: NickWarren557@hotmail.com

isn't it better live, actually doing that stuff?

From: Lori Solomon6697@yahoo.com
you're more attentive to me when you're not actually there with me

From: NickWarren557@hotmail.com
then i guess that's a no

From: Lori Solomon6697@yahoo.com
does it have to be so all or none?

From: NickWarren557@hotmail.com
why not … you like it

The anticipation that encircled their sex-drenched rapport was too tempting to walk away from. Yet the idea of something more tangible or concrete stemming from any of this was daunting. Her passion pit of pure, unadulterated wanton desire was best left as an unmatched fantasy in his mind, the same as his pulsating lightning rod of delight was better off as a remarkable image in hers. Why couldn't she abstain from propositioning him? Why couldn't she just enjoy the ride as a passive spectator?

The next few days brought Lori some reprieve. Her libido was derailed, with school-related stresses causing her to feel drained and weary. She could look at a message from Nick from a distance and not feel powerless to resist the temptation to respond to him. Even her responses carried a careless wit, devoid of the painful gut-kneading emotion she had so often in the past bathed them in. She simply had other things on her mind. And although these things were, in essence, little more than annoying, mundane hassles, she was grateful that they were there to divert her attention away from what she felt was so oddly unsettling.

Chapter 17

Life is just one damned thing after another
Elbert Hubbard (1856-1915)

From: SeriousSchmendrick4428@aol.com
Subject: Entropy
To: LoriSolomon6697@yahoo.com
Lori, do you roll with it? I have begun to roll with it. Whatever it may be at any time that it feels it must be. I acknowledge, I accept, I embrace. I do not become overshadowed by its omnipotence. I instead become one with it. For it is a force meant to guide, not suppress. And I am finding that by being one with that force, I indeed ... am the force. And I am, in essence, my own compass in the seemingly random and directionless realm of being. So I ask again, Lori. Do you roll with it? You're very close, my friend.
Be water....
Rutherford

Lori's energy levels had fallen. She was dragging herself through the long days, and she was falling face-first onto her neglected, squalid bedcovers in the early evenings. She wasn't convinced that only the tiresome hours spent studying were draining her. She believed that it had more to do with the ongoing game of seedy seduction played out like a cat and mouse team in an early Saturday morning kid's cartoon.

Every fifteen to twenty minutes, every day, Lori would walk with Haitian zombie-like glassy eyes to her computer. She would click on the mouse to have the pointer open her e-mail inbox, and she would invariably find two, sometimes three, messages from Nick sent seconds apart from one another. Each harbored the same general adolescent inanity, each was invasively personal, and yet at the same time each was perversely distant.

"Any messages today?" Marta would ask over the phone. Lori could picture her stabbing, smiling blue eyes glaring knowingly on the other end of the receiver. She would wait quietly but anxiously for her fill of vicarious indulgence.

Marta was one of the few people that Lori felt she could discuss her smoky, charcoal black secret with in the absence of any real judgment. Marta had her own demonic possession and war-torn troops of heartless incubi to battle, drawn as she had been to her European versions of the shamelessly unavailable, or just the downright mean. The proverbial nice guy had always been upstaged by the intoxicating power of the elusive in Marta's life, and the beautiful brunette often found herself frustrated and alone.

Time and time again she was sucked into the web of several regular vagabonds in her life, such as the arrogant, commitment-phobic Swiss guy who would periodically toss her a crumb before shoving the whole pie in her face …

"Thanks for taking me out," Marta had said one day in a quaint little outdoor cafe, nudging her hash browns and bacon with her fork.

"Well, I'm just sorry it's been so long since we last did this," Thomas said. "But something just … keeps making me reluctant to approach you. You know? To be with you."

Marta had felt her stomach tighten. "What do you mean?"

He threw his napkin down on his plate. "I don't know," he said, sighing. He wiped his mouth with the back of his hand. "I don't know, Marta."

"What don't you know?" Looking deep into his eyes, she had begun to blindly carve the edges of a poached egg with her butter knife. "What?"

"I …" he started. "I love you."

She blushed and looked down at the sheared egg white on her plate. She pushed the pieces together and started to stack them while she tried to absorb what he had just told her. Her heart had been beating furiously in her chest, her palms beady with sweat.

"But …" he said. "I'm not *in* love with you."

She stared into his eyes again and felt the color drain from her face. She scooped up the napkin that lay on her lap and tossed it down on the table. "Thank you for the brunch," she said, rising to leave. "You may now go and screw yourself."

And there was the shady Internet-obsessed Italian who occasionally surfaced for air like a porpoise before diving deep and out of reach into the sea for weeks or months. Marta would find him "on-line" at all hours of the day, sending and receiving instant messages to and from a myriad of hypothetical girls or guys whose relationships to him would forever remain a mystery to her.

She forwarded a series of instant messenger interactions to Lori.

MatteoS: let's meet
MatteoS: pretty pleaseeeeeeeeeeee
MatteoS: with cherries on top :)
MatteoS: ignoring me?
MartaG: Umm … thought you were pissed at me
MatteoS: i always am. you don't want to meet me
MatteoS: lol
MartaG: I almost forget what you look like?

MatteoS: you know what I look like :) and I sure know what you look like. and smell like :)

MartaG: You're in heat, aren't you?

MatteoS: when I think about you I am :)

MatteoS: not kidding marta

MartaG: Okaaaaaay

MatteoS: ok what?

MatteoS: am I annoying you

MartaG: What do you think?

MartaG: First, you aren't talking to me, and now you are hot for me? What gives?

MatteoS: i asked you out twice and you said you would call but never did

MartaG: That's not how I remember it.

MatteoS: well that is the way it was

MatteoS: i was so looking forward to seeing you again.

MartaG: I had told you that I had a funeral to go to back in Italy. You aren't very understanding

MatteoS: and the time before that?

MartaG: I don't recall a time before that

MatteoS: anyway. i have to admit i miss you. a lot

MartaG: Are you pulling my leg?

MatteoS: no marta

MatteoS: i get all hot and steamy just thinking about how well we kiss together

MatteoS: but you know that already

MartaG: Well, ya!

MatteoS: but it is like pulling teeth trying to hook up with you

MartaG: Deep down I miss you too, but can't just see each other in person twice a year!

MartaG: Don't you ever crave more?

MartaG: Matteo?

MartaG: Matteo? Are you still there?

After apparently not putting out to Matteo's satisfaction one evening because Marta claimed she needed time to get to know him better as a person, he began avoiding her by not sending her his usual instant messages at times when she could plainly see that he was "on line." Then one special evening, the silence broke with an expression of concern on Matteo's part over not having heard from Marta for so long. His heartfelt display of attention and sincerity was immediately followed by a request to see her again. Marta realized that perhaps it was *she* who wronged *him*. Perhaps she wasn't as available to him as she could have been, or should have been. She eagerly accepted his invitation, and then found herself twiddling her thumbs alone in her apartment and staring angrily at her quiet phone on the Tuesday night they were tentatively scheduled to see one another. Then she faced another month or so of Internet silence before Matteo returned once more to ask her point blank in an instant message why she "blew him off." Her reply was that she was heavily engrossed in filing her nails and she would appreciate it if he would go screw himself.

Whereas Marta's reasons for being innkeeper of her own Moron Motel were unclear, Lori believed that the darkness she herself was drawn to may have been some kind of an attempt to conquer a modern-day reincarnation of lost tainted loves and old-time bullies. Nick Warren seemed to be the Hell-selected envoy of everything in her life that had gone wrong, everything in her life she never forgave herself for allowing to go wrong. Nothing came closer to the truth than her friend Angela's drunkenly spewed philosophy to Natalie on that one grim New Year's eve: "You've got to stop letting the dickheads run and ruin your life. You keep inviting the dickheads in; I keep inviting the dickheads in. 'Cause they remind us of all those other dickheads who were there before them. And we think we can change them and we try to change them because we never had the chance to change the other dickheads and by having a new dickhead to change we're being given another chance."

She started to read a message from Rutherford.

From: SeriousSchmendrick4428@aol.com
Subject: foot odor
To: LoriSolomon6697@yahoo.com
"Woe to them be that not believe, for thy bed be waft with a foul pox; no light doth hath them for a road when cleaved in twain, an enemy of God, nor a fixture bearing the hands of angels shall be the place to set their towels when damp."
What do you think? For the last couple of days I've been reading the Bible and the Koran ... and I've concluded that as long as you write stuff with weird words like "hath" and "thou" and "doth," you're bound to get some followers. In a word, I'm thinking of founding a new religion. I just need to find a group of people to hate. Hatred is an interesting theme in these books, incidentally. In the Bible, the Egyptians and the Romans are the bad guys, and in the Koran you only have to read about two pages before it mentions that the Jews are wicked.
"Woe be it to the children born of the foot of the Alps, for they are unbelievers, and doth barter a wedge of raclette for twice the market price and giggle. God hates them for this!"
Let me know if you want to join my cult...
Rutherford

Lori's phone rang.
"Hey. It's me."

"Hey," Lori said.

"What are you doing now?"

"Studying."

"Did you get my last e-mail?" Nick asked.

"No. I haven't had the chance to check. Why? What does it say?"

"Read it," he said.

"Okay."

"Guess I better let you get back to studying now," he said.

"All right."

"Bye." He quickly hung up the phone.

From: Nick Warren
u warm?

Lori stared long and hard at his message, just one of the many hollow, echoing cries of superficiality that she found herself completely unable to ignore. She wondered when this was all going to come to an end. And she wondered how she would feel when, in fact, it finally did.

From: Lori Solomon6697@yahoo.com
for THIS you called me?

From: NickWarren557@hotmail.com
yeah i wanted to know if u were getting warm?

Lori paused. She knew that this would only come to an end when she made it come to an end. Yet what kind of an ending did she want? How was she going to make it happen? More importantly, did she really *want* it to happen? Did she really want it to end?

Chapter 18

It's not true that life is one damn thing after another; it is one damn thing over and over
Edna St. Vincent Millay (1892-1950)

From: AngelontheAirwaves3254@hotmail.com
Subject: Re:
To: LoriSolomon6697@yahoo.com
So I had to tell my Ayurvedic guide that I can't continue my 70-dollar sessions with her. I do have a referral from my doctor for a counselor who's on my insurance plan. She's a licensed clinical social worker, as opposed to a doctor. The co-pays would only be 20 dollars. Sessions are limited, though.

From: LoriSolomon6697@yahoo.com
Subject: Re:
To: AngelontheAirwaves3254@hotmail.com
Sounds good. It's a start. Too bad you can't continue with your Ayurvedic guide, though. Speaking of which, I still need to get those colonic cleansers she had suggested to you.

From: AngelontheAirwaves3254@hotmail.com
Subject: Re:
To: LoriSolomon6697@yahoo.com
They are just called colon cleansers, not colonic. Is that even a word? I think I sent you a website where you could get them, didn't I?
Angela

From: LoriSolomon6697@yahoo.com
Subject: Re:
To: AngelontheAirwaves3254@hotmail.com

Oxygen Colonic Cleanser... There's also Colonic Cleanser Dietary Oxygen Supplement. Don't know if it's the same thing as what your Ayurvedic guide suggested, but "colonic" is obviously a word.
Lori

From: AngelontheAirwaves3254@hotmail.com
Subject: Re:
To: LoriSolomon6697@yahoo.com
I STAND CORRECTED. BITCH.

From: LoriSolomon6697@yahoo.com
Subject: Re:
To: AngelontheAirwaves3254@hotmail.com
Did you ever just feel like you're sitting in place, just spinning your wheels? That's how I've been feeling, Angela, for a long time now ... With college... Science … Broadcasting … It's like, all this work, and all this running around ... what's the point? Where am I GOING with all this?

From: AngelontheAirwaves3254@hotmail.com
Subject: Re:
To: LoriSolomon6697@yahoo.com
You have NOT been "spinning your wheels." Would you PLEASE stop talking like that? You accomplish something every bloody day.

From: LoriSolomon6697@yahoo.com
Subject: Re:
To: AngelontheAirwaves3254@hotmail.com
Like Paul always used to say, I'm one of those "perpetually dissatisfied" people. Guess it's a pathology of sorts. I just always feel like whatever I'm doing just isn't enough. I don't know why I feel this way, but I swear it's something that I always carry around with me.

Maybe I have too many things in life that I'd like to accomplish and experience, and I feel like I haven't even scraped the surface.

From: AngelontheAirwaves3254@hotmail.com
Subject: Re:
To: LoriSolomon6697@yahoo.com
See, Lori, here's the problem with your self-acknowledged "pathology" (and I do think you are correct in your assessment). When you talk or write to me about how much you think you still need to accomplish, it fills me with a sense of discomfort. It makes me feel very uneasy, because I get to thinking, "Damn, if she doesn't think she's accomplished enough, what can she possibly think of ME???" And it really clashes with MY insecurities that "I'm never good enough." So I'm just sharing that with you so that you will know how your "issues" might negatively affect someone else. It's the same when you chastise yourself for gaining weight and reaching 125-130 pounds, when you know that I'm pushing 180. Know what I mean?
Angela

From: LoriSolomon6697@yahoo.com
Subject: Re:
To: AngelontheAirwaves3254@hotmail.com
Angela, as much as I understand what you're saying, I really think you need to do some serious work on your own insecurities. You internalize a lot of what other people say or do and make it about you. That's doing your own self a disservice. I don't think about you when I'm thinking about myself. I'm just concentrating on the things that I want out of life. Has absolutely nothing to do with you or what you've done with your life. I figure, how can we even compare? And why would we want

to? We've been leading separate lives, focusing on different things.

From: AngelontheAirwaves3254@hotmail.com
Subject: Re:
To: LoriSolomon6697@yahoo.com
Oh, I know, I know. You are completely right! That's why I made a point to say that sometimes your "pathology" (or whatever you want to call it) clashes with mine. I know I take everything personally and allow myself to feel inferior way too easily. I honestly do take responsibility for that.
That having been said, I need to tell you as a friend (the way Paul would) that if you do not "lighten up" on yourself, you are going to end up with some health problem that could at worst have the effect of keeping you from fulfilling any goal. Not trying to scare you, but I've seen it happen to too many people who are over-achievers. They end up making themselves so sick that they can't achieve anything.
Life is meant to be enjoyed, Lori. You don't need to be contributing to the world every minute of every day. It's not healthy. It's not fair to you or the people around you when you drive yourself so hard. That's me being objective. I care about you. Stop. Relax. Smell the roses.
Angela

Lori decided to take the last two days of the workweek off from going to her classes. Her head was spinning in a cloud of turmoil, her heart as brittle as a sheet of hardened peanut-strewn molasses. If she did not break away, just for a short while, she was sure she would go mad.
Sitting on her living room couch in her little Springfield apartment on a late Thursday morning

reminded Lori of being in a secluded cabin retreat in the middle of dense forest in mountainous terrain. She was alone with nothing but the sound of a clock ticking on a fireplace mantel, nothing but a stale box of crackers from the Neolithic Period she had pulled from the dark, webbed recesses of her kitchen cabinet, nothing but a pile of press releases on her coffee table.

She lifted the stack of articles high over her head, relishing the feeling of blood rushing fast down the lengths of her arms. She set the press releases down in front of her, and positioned an empty notepad next to them. She knew that although she was getting closer to what the radio station's program coordinator wanted in terms of sounding more like a journalist, she still had a distance to go before he would consider using any of her work. She figured that all she needed were one or two solid days of uninterrupted concentration on the task at hand to bring her closer to success.

She needed to completely detach herself. She glanced carelessly at the shadowy doorway of her bedroom, and then shifted her eyes to the empty hallway just outside of it. She had hours and hours of solitude laid out before her like a scrumptious all-you-can-eat buffet.

She waited until late evening to take her first break from her work. She stood up, stretched her tightened back muscles, and casually meandered past her bedroom door and toward her dark, idle PC. While she waited for the computer to warm up, she could almost count down to the exact second when her gut would start to spasm with fluttering winged creatures bouncing off its walls. The mild euphoria she was beginning to feel from being quarantined for hours instantly waned once her fingers began pressing her personal e-mail code on the computer keys. The number "1" sat in her inbox. As she positioned the little pointing animated hand over the inbox, she worried that it was an Internet advertisement for a free camera or cell phone, or worse, an impersonal forwarded group message from her uncle Hyman.

It was Rutherford. It was a message that he had sent to her the previous night.

From: SeriousSchmendrick4428@aol.com
Subject: Chipotle Rib Extravaganza!
To: LoriSolomon6697@yahoo.com
My "world" you asked, is one of ritual, foolishness, and boredom. I'm still obsessed with mastering Pac Man, and yet with all my progress and practice I still have yet to get a score better than 250,000. This game is driving me insane! All that matters in life is Pac Man, Lori. It's a perfect metaphor for our worthless existences as well: The Pac Man guy is each of us; the "ghosts" are our obstacles to avoid and therefore overcome; the power-dots are our moments of inspiration and invincibility that get shorter and shorter as the game lags on; the "bonus fruits" are our meager rewards for our efforts; and ultimately we will always lose and DIE without beating the system.
I can't think of any other video game that is so reflective of the way the real world works.
Either way, I'm just bored and tired with it all.
Rutherford

From: LoriSolomon6697@yahoo.com
Subject: Re:
To: SeriousSchmendrick4428@aol.com
I suppose in my own way, I'm "bored" and "tired" of it all, too. I stayed home today to try to regain some momentum. I've been feeling really drained lately. I've

been exhausted, and at the same time I can't seem to get enough sleep.

I just have this kind of dull feeling. I don't know what it is or where it's coming from. Maybe it's a slow, subtle descent into incurable insanity. I don't know. All I know is that I feel "dull."

Lori

From: SeriousSchmendrick4428@aol.com
Subject: Rib Extravaganza!
To: LoriSolomon6697@yahoo.com

I understand what you mean about feeling "dull." There's nothing worse than an overwhelming sense of dullness in life. That "sharp" versus "dull" metaphor is a great one. Life just seems to have no "edge" sometimes ... It's worse than a dull knife. Have you ever tried to slice a really juicy, ripe tomato with a dull knife? Believe me, it's a nightmare.

Listen, my darling, you need to EMBRACE your free time; utilize it for creative purposes; learn how to stare at the wall for 3 or 4 hours without thinking about ANYTHING; consider the astronomical implications of the God-vs-Human-vs-Nature dynamic ... ANYTHING. The reason you get "depressed" is because you're uncomfortable with any lifestyle that isn't pre-ordered, controlled, and easily predicted. Do you follow? Right now, you're a slave to expectations that everyone ELSE has of you, rather than following your own true path. Tell me I'm wrong, dammit, you KNOW I'm right! You're well on your way to becoming a wild-woman stuck in a laboratory frock.... A free spirit aching for release...

Rutherford (a.k.a. Scalp Man)

From: LoriSolomon6697@yahoo.com
Subject: Re:
To: SeriousSchmendrick4428@aol.com

Sometimes it's a blessing to be alone because you can appreciate life in an undistracted kind of way that you otherwise couldn't. I remember having plenty of "alone" moments back in high school that I still to this day look back on. I actually felt for a long time that my high school days were my "glory days"—mostly because I really didn't MIND all those times being alone.
Lori

From: SeriousSchmendrick4428@aol.com
Subject: Extravaganza!
To: LoriSolomon6697@yahoo.com
Deary-dear,
Being "alone" is the best thing that ever happened to me. It may sound strange, but I'm so glad that I didn't grow up surrounded by friends/lovers/DISTRACTIONS you wouldn't believe it. When I was a punk-ass adolescent and then a teenager, I was rather ugly and unattractive (huh? Are those separate things?), so I found myself alone almost ALL the time. At that age, I was miserable because I thought the key to life was connecting with people. But I quickly learned how to simply ACCEPT being alone and actually use it to my advantage. Now, I actually PREFER to be alone, and I think my track record with girls in particular supports that. I've decided that I LIKE being alone. Leave me alone!
Interestingly enough, did you know that the word "alone" is a conjunction of the words "all" and "one"? Think about it... ALL ONE = ALONE. The term "alone" was invented to explain the wholeness that a single individual feels even though she/he is seemingly separate from everyone else. I'm not making this up, Lori. You can look it up if you want. It's another historical thingie that makes beautiful sense when you think about it.

Oh well, whatever. Tonight, I plan to finally break 300,000 on Pac Man. Wish me luck…
Rutherford (a.k.a. The Danish-Irish-Buddhist-Taoist-Pantheist-Orthodox dork)

Perhaps all Lori needed was to continue embracing her solitude to feel whole again. After all, it seemed as though the vast majority of the distress she felt at any point in her life could usually be traced to some*one* as opposed to some*thing*. It was possible that keeping herself a safe distance away from everything for just a few more hours, for just one more day, was enough to infuse her with the strength she needed.

She awakened the following morning feeling apprehensive. While she waited for a mug of instant cocoa to heat up in her microwave oven, she eased off of a twisted heap of blanket and slid into the chair in front of her computer. She stared owl-eyed as the computer screen slowly developed, barely conscious of the microwave beeping in the kitchen down the hall.

From: Lori Solomon6697@yahoo.com
i'm going to be home all day. i'll be checking my messages throughout, if you want to keep "in touch"
Lori

She grabbed her mug of steaming cocoa, hoisted her loose pajama bottoms up around her waist and walked over to her living room couch. She started perusing unread press releases. Clutching her drink, she read them over until she began reading over the same lines without grasping their meaning. She soon meandered back into her bedroom and sat cross-legged on the chair in front of her computer.

From: NickWarren557@hotmail.com

WELL I WISH I COULD COME RIGHT OVER AND ...
YOUR LOVE BOX.

She smiled at the thought that this was the closest Nick had ever come to using the word "love" in reference to her. As she sipped the thin layer of lukewarm foam off of the surface of her hot chocolate, she wondered if Nick was truly capable of loving someone. She wondered if he was truly capable of caring about someone. She wondered if he was truly capable of *liking* someone, unconditionally.

From: Nick Warren557@hotmail.com
PLEASE TELL ME WHAT YOU ARE WEARING.

From: Lori Solomon6697@yahoo.com
satin bikini underwear and a sports bra

She glanced down at her coffee-stained, oversized white t-shirt and men's pajamas with an unattractive plaid print design and open crotch flap. She took another sip of her cocoa, this time burning the tip of her tongue on the lava-like liquid.

From: Nick Warren557@hotmail.com
WOW!!!

From: Lori Solomon6697@yahoo.com
could you call me later?

From: Nick Warren557@hotmail.com
I'M AT WORK SO I CAN'T CALL AND SAY THINGS LIKE WHAT I WANT TO...

From: Lori Solomon6697@yahoo.com
can't you call after work?

From: Nick Warren557@hotmail.com
WELL I CAN BUT REMEMBER I LIVE WITH MONA
STILL AND ITS TOUGH TO CALL WHEN SHE IS
HOME ... BUT THE SNEAKINESS MAKES IT MORE
EXCITING!

She knew that she had no right to feel anything
after reading what he had just written to her.
Nonetheless, she felt as though she had a 105° fever
and someone had just taken an ice cube and rubbed it
against the small of her back. She stood up, stretched
her legs, and walked back into her living room with the
intention of trying to escape into more press releases.
She lifted up a page on stem cell research, glared at it
for several seconds, and then placed it back down on a
large stack of untouched reports. She skulked back into
her bedroom, sat down at the keyboard, and bit her
lower lip until it started to sting as much as her tongue.

From: Lori Solomon6697@yahoo.com
you're back with Mona???!!!

From: Nick Warren557@hotmail.com
I HAVE BEEN FOR A WHILE. I THOUGHT I TOLD
YOU...

From: Lori Solomon6697@yahoo.com
the last time i talked to you was at the launch party
you told me she wanted to be alone

From: Nick Warren557@hotmail.com
YEAH THAT WAS A WHILE AGO

From: Lori Solomon6697@yahoo.com
so what's the story with you two

From: Nick Warren557@hotmail.com
she lives with me … dating i guess … that is what is up

From: Lori Solomon 6697@yahoo.com
live-in "playmates?"

From: Nick Warren557@hotmail.com
yeah i guess you can say that … i like playmates

From: Lori Solomon6697@yahoo.com
you don't feel like you're hurting her by going behind her back?

From: Nick Warren557@hotmail.com
well what about your situation … with paul?

From: Lori Solomon6697@yahoo.com
i don't know

From: Lori Solomon6697@yahoo.com
am i turning into your secret playmate?

From: Nick Warren557@hotmail.com
yes you are…. is that a problem

From: Lori Solomon6697@yahoo.com
no
that's what i want

In truth, she had no idea what she wanted. And this was partly because she had no idea what he wanted. That is, if he truly wanted anything at all.

As for Paul, she hadn't spoken to him since the night of the radioactive spill during her internship in the *Drosophila* lab. Shaken, the shrill sound of the activated

Geiger counter still resonating in her ears long after she had left the scene, she had thought of Paul as the only person who always seemed to know just what to say to her to calm her. She recalled the relief she had felt upon hearing his voice on the other end of the phone.

"It'll be okay," he had said. "You have to remember that the half-life of P32 is really short. Even if you can't get all of it up tonight, it'll be gone before you know it."

She couldn't stop sobbing into the phone. "I'm going to get pregnant some day and give birth to a three-headed monster with ten legs!"

"Lori, trust me. As nasty as the stuff is, the spill could've been a lot worse if you were using something like tritium, which hangs around forever. And you *found* the contamination. Think about what would've happened if it went undetected."

She walked into the bathroom and started to fill her tub with hot, sudsy water. She sat Indian-style on the bath mat with her fingers clutching the rim, and watched the bubbly surface creep slowly up the rusty porcelain walls. She stood up and dipped one foot in at a time. She hoped that all would come clear as the astronomical temperature anesthetized her skin and calmed her.

She was soon lost in the fragrant mist of serenity that filled the thick, heated air. After a while, she stood up and wrapped a clean, soft towel around herself. Trailing water and soapsuds across the hardwood floor of the narrow hallway leading into her bedroom, she felt relaxed enough to continue.

From: Lori Solomon6697@yahoo.com
are we done for the day, playmate?

From: Nick Warren557@hotmail.com

maybe

From: Lori Solomon6697@yahoo.com
has the moment of excitement for you passed?

From: Nick Warren557@hotmail.com
no

Lori roamed away again from the computer. She sat herself down in the middle of her living room couch, and began pouring over press releases and siphoning out those she thought would be interesting to broadcast. It was only when she felt as though she had gotten a decent amount done that she wandered back to the computer.

From: Lori Solomon6697@yahoo.com
months ago you told me you wanted to commit to Mona what changed?

From: Nick Warren557@hotmail.com
ahh i dunno. its just me i guess. i like lots of different kinds to choose from

From: Lori Solomon6697@yahoo.com
does she know this?

From: Nick Warren557@hotmail.com
no.... oh well

From: Lori Solomon6697@yahoo.com
you complained a while back that she cheated on you that upset you, right?

From: Nick Warren557@hotmail.com
yeah ... oh well

From: Lori Solomon6697@yahoo.com
you don't seem to care too much one way or the other,
do you?

From: Nick Warren557@hotmail.com
i guess
lol … hehe
you cant get enough of me.

From: Lori Solomon6697@yahoo.com
and you can't get enough of me
am i right?

From: Nick Warren557@hotmail.com
maybe … i have something you like and need and you
have something that i like and need … so it seems that
we help each other out in some way

From: Lori Solomon6697@yahoo.com
is there something more that i'm giving you?

From: Nick Warren557@hotmail.com
no i have shown the open doors to you of things that
can be done differently and excitement

Lori sat back in her chair. Perhaps he typed faster
than his thoughts came to mind, or perhaps he barely
put any thought into his messages at all. Whatever the
problem was, Lori often had as much difficulty trying to
understand what he was writing as she did trying to
understand the broken English of Pista Bakfark.

From: Lori Solomon6697@yahoo.com
so what do you "need" from me?

From: Nick Warren557@hotmail.com
just what i have been after!

From: Lori Solomon6697@yahoo.com
but you've had me in the past
you're not tired of it?

From: Nick Warren557@hotmail.com
no ...

Chapter 19

Rejoice not at thine enemy's fall- but don't rush to pick him up either
Jewish Proverb

From: AngelontheAirwaves3254@hotmail.com
Subject: Re:
To: LoriSolomon6697@yahoo.com
I wanted you to know that I e-mailed Rutherford and I got a very nice e-mail back. We're on the friendship track again. I actually wasn't even expecting a response from him, and the good news is I didn't care one way or another (that's how over him I am). But when he DID respond, I was happy. I just cannot care too much about how much he decides to mess up his life. I am learning to become detached from the outcomes of everything.
At the same time, my mother was literally screaming at the top of her lungs at me when I told her I was back in touch with him. She thinks I'm headed for a big fall, and she doesn't understand why I don't just leave well enough alone and accept the fact that he and I don't get along and just get on with my life.
Angela

From: LoriSolomon6697@yahoo.com
Subject: Re:
To: AngelontheAirwaves3254@hotmail.com
Angela, whenever you make choices that inevitably end up being bad- for whatever reason- the outcome and impact doesn't just affect you. It affects those who are closest to you at the time (your parents, your friends). And your parents are getting older. They're the ones you lean on the most, and it can be exhausting for them, not to mention frustrating. I think your family feels

that if you could make choices in your life that are sound and well thought out and that put you at least risk of getting hurt, they'll worry less about you, and any impact your choices may eventually have on THEM. Does this make sense to you? Your living situation coupled with your tendency to have very strong reactions to things, are such that your parents are directly intertwined in your life. And they suffer when you suffer. Maybe even more so.

Lori

From: AngelontheAirwaves3254@hotmail.com
Subject: Re:
To: LoriSolomon6697@yahoo.com

I agree with all that you have said about my parents. And I understand completely how the decisions that I make, good or bad, inevitably affect them and other people who care about me. That having been said, I think my parents were very instrumental in some of the "bad" ways I developed emotionally. I haven't had a chance to share this with you yet (perhaps we can talk tonight), but I had a HUGE fight with my father Friday night, after which he was giving me three months to "get the hell" out of "his" house. It was brutal, the worst we've ever had. It was triggered when he couldn't stop gushing about how "beautiful" my kid sister, Jamie, looked, before going to her very first dance. He kept saying, "She is beautiful, absolutely gorgeous," and on and on and on. Suddenly, from the very depths of my soul, I was agonizingly reminded of all the positive reinforcement I DID NOT GET FROM HIM WHILE GROWING UP. And, in fact, I was told that I was decidedly NOT beautiful, never would be, and I just needed to accept that and move on. Now, you tell me, Lori, what child of adolescent age could possibly want to hear that from her beloved father? I don't give a rat's ass if the bastard had to LIE to me. HE SHOULD HAVE TOLD ME THAT, IN HIS EYES, I WAS INDEED BEAUTIFUL, AND TO HELL WITH THE MORONS AT SCHOOL WHO WERE TELLING ME OTHERWISE.

But understand my anger was not just about what my father had denied me with regard to my physical appearance. It was also the general lack of emotional support for nearly everything I'd ever gone through in my youth- from peer issues, to boys, to friendships. He NEVER seemed to validate my feelings about ANYTHING, instead always making me feel like my feelings were silly and stupid. And later in life, he'd think nothing of telling me I was "sick" in the head.

Add to that, the crappy way I always saw him treat my mother, so intimidating, and verbally abusive ... and you have the victim- that would be ME- of a pretty dysfunctional upbringing. If my childhood had been one bit better, it's quite possible that I would have learned to make much more intelligent, rational decisions with regard to the guys I allow close to me. It's easy to say, "Take responsibility for your life NOW and just get over it." But it's a whole lot more difficult to "just get over" something that has insidiously eaten away at your very soul for your whole life. In fact, it may even be impossible. Feelings of inferiority and not being "good enough" are so indelibly etched in my brain ... I fear I may never be able to undo them...

Angela

Lori woke up in the morning to find an avalanche of messages on the computer from Nick. She would have been flattered by this sudden unsolicited attention had she not become conditioned over time to suspect pure selfish motive as the driving force behind his actions.

From: Nick Warren557@hotmail.com
HEY HUNNY IT'S NICK HERE

From: Nick Warren557@hotmail.com
so did you miss me??

From: Nick Warren557@hotmail.com
hey i called you last night … got machine twice

From: Lori Solomon6697@yahoo.com
i was at the radio station voicing science reports until midnight
where was Mona?

From: Nick Warren557@hotmail.com
ahh should have called me. we could have done things. hott things

From: Lori Solomon6697@yahoo.com
where wuzzzzzzzzzzz mooooooonaaaaaa??????!!!!

From: Nick Warren557@hotmail.com
i dunno

Lori stopped typing. She felt sorry for him. Although she had no idea how oddly or badly he behaved behind the closed doors of his daddy's basement, where he and Mona were living together, it was clear that he habitually found himself deserted by his young live-in lover. She found that she was more intrigued, and in some ways saddened, by this strange on-again, off-again affair of his than she was by their own peculiar on-again, off-again relationship. She would have given almost anything to be a cognizant fly on a wall in his abode, to see what weakness hid beneath the veil of bravado. All the same, she wondered if she really needed to burden herself with the pursuit of someone else's mystery, as she was still trying hard to uncover her own.

Over the next week, she was inundated with talk so outrageously perverted and graphic it could make a triple X porn star wince and shyly curl up in a fetal position. She wasn't sure if she was finding herself more fascinated by the sheer absurdity of what Nick was churning out, or by his shocking millisecond delay promptness in responding to everything she sent to him. For a solid week, she was his submissive beast of burden, racing back and forth to and from her home computer twenty or more times a day to respond to his conscienceless streams-of-consciousness. She felt herself becoming more and more defiled with every click of every button on the computer keypad, and yet she was completely powerless to stop.

For so long she had tried to purge herself of the queer, untoward preoccupation she had with this oversexed, overgrown child, and yet she was emerging from her futile struggle even more dishearteningly obsessive than when she had begun it. For every moment in time that she had thought of and desired him over the time she had known him, she secretly wished for him to think of and desire her. And so now, being on his mind throughout each and every day for a solid month and a half-- even if it was mainly in the form of a large, floating, accommodating orifice-- was truly a psychotic's dream come true.

From: Nick Warren557@hotmail.com
hey cum over tonight. call me later on my cell phone

From: Lori Solomon6697@yahoo.com

i have hours … and hours … and HOURS of studying to do tonight…

From: Nick Warren557@hotmail.com
tomorrow night??? i will make you ...

From: Lori Solomon6697@yahoo.com
it's got to be another night
where's Mona?

From: Nick Warren557@hotmail.com
she does what she wants and i do whats i want …

From: Lori Solomon6697@yahoo.com
so did you and Mona split?

From: Nick Warren557@hotmail.com
yeah we sorta split … so she wont be there …
so what do you want me to do to you? tell me in detail!!!!

It was decided that they would meet the following Monday night at the Belchertown radio station. Lori impatiently drove her car that evening along the snaking country road that led to the old, dilapidated building. She pushed hard on the gas pedal, and noticed that her legs felt the same heaviness and numbness that they would otherwise feel right before she had to stand up and give an oral presentation for one of her classes. She felt her heart thumping hard and fast within her chest, and she was finding it difficult to catch her breath. Having done so often in the past the same foolish thing she was about to do, she knew she was putting a bounty on her very own head, and would soon be paying a heavy emotional fine for her lack of restraint, yet again.

An old familiar purple Chevrolet and white minivan sat in the station's private parking lot, yet there was also an off-white Honda that Lori had never before seen. She stepped out of her car to round the far corner of the building to see if Nick's fire engine red Thunderbird was hiding beneath two imposing Satellite dishes planted in the station's backyard. The rear of the dark establishment was vacant, although she wondered if perhaps Nick had switched vehicles in the time that had gone by since she had last seen his trademark crimson muscle car.

Faint sounds of Brazilian music emanating from the second floor suggested that someone was busy playing Spanish disc jockey in one of the upstairs studios. Figuring that perhaps Nick might have been waiting for her inside as well, she stepped into the tiny front corridor of the station and peered through the glass of the inner door. There was no one in her immediate view, although the door suddenly buzzed loudly and opened up, allowing her to step inside the building.

She peered down the main, narrow hallway and began to search all dark and dank levels of the station for signs of human life. The Brazilian music continued to vibrate the walls from a small, secluded studio at the top of a staircase. She figured that this was the only room in the entire house that was occupied.

She walked back to the front doorway and stood there, peering out into the warm, breezy night. The same vehicles she had seen earlier flanked her own in the parking lot, and any new cars coming into the vicinity of the station merely flashed their blinding headlights for a second in her direction before continuing to fly by on the busy nearby thoroughfare.

She walked outside again, quietly climbed back inside her car, and stuck her key into the ignition. She was about to leave when she heard the sound of an engine grow louder as a car turned from the road into the parking lot and pulled itself into a vacant space by the minivan. She started to breathe heavily and she felt the muscles in her thighs tighten as though she had just died and rigor mortis was setting in. She opened her car door, still sitting and facing forward, still clutching her car key and keeping it in place inside the ignition slot. In her periphery, she saw a figure emerging from the car. Out of the corner of her eye, she saw the figure walking behind the minivan toward her.

"I was just about to go," she said quietly. She stared up at the figure.

Nick stood with his hands in his pockets a few feet away from her. Despite his strange, unkempt Unabomber look, with a long, bushy ZZ-Top beard and wild, wavy dark hair, she could still manage to find the boy behind the beast that made her heart race.

"Why?" he asked, softly.

"I'm nervous," she said, stepping outside of her car.

"But why?" he asked again. He drew himself near to where she stood and leaned his back against her car. He placed his hands on her waist and lifted her shirt to see and touch what lay underneath. Then he pulled her close so he could kiss her hard on her lips and grab at her rear.

"Come on. Let's go," he said. He motioned for her to join him for a ride to his daddy's house. She sat down in his fur-lined passenger bucket seat and said as little as she could while he took her on a tour of several residential neighborhoods many miles away from the station. She was afraid to open her mouth and say anything, a post-traumatic stress reaction to the last time that she was alone in a car with him. She sat in silence and forced him to fill the uncomfortable void with whatever shallow topics he was able to come up with. She wondered how she could feel so drawn to someone she was so frightened of, and what the pathology was that lay beneath her need to repeatedly place herself in harm's way.

A fluffy white cat raced out of his home and toward the car when they arrived. Only seconds after Lori stepped up onto the front porch leading into the house, she was guided through an open door leading away from what appeared to be papa's kitchen, and down into the basement. A dirty welcome mat greeted her at the base of the stairwell, and she smiled at the irony of its existence in the home of someone she would hesitate to label as typically "congenial." Behind a large, covered pool table sat a small brown dresser with a plastic box filled with hair ornaments and picks sitting on top of it.

"See? Mona's still got some of her stuff here," he said, pointing to what Lori had already figured out was hers. It seemed important to him for Lori to know that she did, indeed, exist in his world.

"Where is she?" Lori asked. She sat down on a plush off-white couch encircling a big screen television set.

"She's been workin' at a hotel. They're letting her sleep there." He ran up the stairs to fetch "cheap beer" that he thought his father had stored in their refrigerator. He returned seconds later with one can and one bottle of ale for the two of them.

"Would you like to see my room?" he asked.

Lori stood up, clutching her unopened, frosty beer can. She walked into a small alcove. The floor was almost completely covered by a queen-sized bed decorated with a dark blue comforter and many soft, full pillows. Another television set sat on a black dresser near the doorway, and Grateful Dead posters filled almost every inch of wall space.

"What is that?" she asked, pointing to two strips of brown and white fur nailed into one of the few free patches of wall adjacent to his bed.

"It's an animal," he said obscurely. He reached for her jeans and tugged at them until they dropped to the floor. She stepped outside of the masses of wrinkled denim and was surprised to find him taking the care to pull her socks off of her feet, one by one.

As they frolicked, with daddy sleeping only feet away in an upstairs bedroom, Nick seemed much more attentive to her than he had been months earlier. He was pleasant, patient, almost tinkering on the edge of being sweet, although still in a rough and tumbled back street boy kind of way.

"Can I put my arm around you?" Lori asked, as he lay on his side next to her on the bed.

"Yeah. I'm right here," he responded coolly, continuing to balance his weight on one elbow as he stared at her body from several inches away. "Go ahead."

She placed her left arm under his torso, wanting to pull him close, yet unable to do much more than touch his bare skin with her own. Nick had just seen heaven moments earlier, and now it was her turn to do the same. Yet what he didn't seem to realize was that anything and everything that Lori needed to taste forbidden paradise was the complete opposite of what he apparently thought she needed. Or the complete opposite of what he was willing to let her have.

"Pretend I'm on the phone," he said, suddenly, sitting up and leaning over her. With closed eyes, she reached for his leg and felt him jerk it away. "Pretend I'm not here. I'm not here. I'm just a voice. There's no one here but you. You ... and ... two guys. Just you

215

and two guys. Brad Pitt and Tom Cruise, climbing all over you."

"Are you there, too, with me?" she asked.

"No," he said.

"But you're the only one I want in the fantasy," she said. "I don't know the other two … I don't care about the other two."

"O.K., O.K.," he said, frantically. "I'm there. In the fantasy."

Lori opened her eyes just long enough to watch him do a little jig while stark naked near the edge of his bed. "How's this? Does this get you excited?" he asked as he shook his shoulders and wiggled his hips and caused every free chest hair and dangling appendage to sway in rhythm right along with him.

Lori sat up in his bed and started gathering her clothes. "I think I'm done," she said gently.

"What?" he asked.

"There's … too much pressure," she said, smiling. "I'll be all right. Don't worry."

They began driving back to the radio station. Again, she sat in near silence as he struggled for things to say to ward off the gaps in the conversation. She responded only to subjects that he brought up, making sure to make her statements as brief and to the point as their e-mail messages to one another had always been. She felt that this was the only type of communication that Nick could handle, as anything more layered would bore or disturb him. Or bring him too close. Her most revealing gesture was the presentation of a newspaper clipping of an anticancer drug her brother had been working on. After a brief explanation of what it was, she set the folded article down behind the gearbox.

"O.K., hun," he said. He drove into the lot and pulled up next to her car. He shifted into the parked position and turned to face her, but she had already opened the passenger side door and placed one leg outside and onto the pavement. In a quick fit of latent revenge, she tried to run away from him almost as callously as he had run away from her months ago. Yet she could only be so heartless. She softly said "good-night" to him as she pulled her other leg outside and set her foot on the ground.

"I'll read this," he called to her, holding up her brother's article. "But honestly, I'm really just into reading about stuff having to do with my own condition."

His condition. She often forgot about it, since it wasn't a subject that had come up again between the two of them since the day she met him. Then again, there weren't many subjects that tended to come up between them, even though they could find themselves interacting conservatively seventy or eighty times a day for stretches of weeks at a time.

She had difficulty seeing the lock of her car in the shadowy darkness, and she hunched over it for several seconds, cursing under her breath and trying to get the key to slide into it. She noticed that Nick was still sitting in his car, very possibly chivalrously waiting for her to get the door ajar before he slowly pulled his car out of the lot.

Lori drove home without so much as turning on the radio, feeling nothing in particular. It may have been little more than fatigue draining her of her ability to feel any real, solid emotion. Yet it may have been the sputtering, wheezing finale of weeks and weeks of steady and steamy libidinous build-up. Build-up that was predicted to be followed by even more of an anticlimactic thud, were Nick to follow his old time love'em and leave 'em tradition.

She knew they were nothing to each other but sex. What held them together was so primitive, so raw, that it made just about any demeaning, demoralizing, or dehumanizing behavior on either of their parts completely excusable. Removing him from her life, if that was what she decided to do, would actually be quite easy. All she had to do was stop pursuing or responding to him. He'd eventually go away. But getting him out of her mind was something that would take considerably more strength. Perhaps a certain degree of genius.

The pure, dense, black and white reasoning Lori knew from when she was a child had somehow over the years turned gray and pixilated. She thought she knew what she needed to get through life, to get through life in a "path of least resistance" kind of way. Yet there was also the question of what she *wanted*. What she believed she wanted was not at all the same thing as what she needed. What she believed she needed seemed to be all she was expected to have. And all she was expected to have just didn't seem to be enough.

She wondered how her cravings got to be so complex, so difficult to fulfill in a simple, straightforward way. Whether it was what she was doing or whom she was doing, she seemed to have the same forces tugging at her in opposing directions. She wanted serenity and stability, yet she didn't want boredom. She wanted mystery and excitement, yet she didn't want trouble. She wanted to live her life like there was no tomorrow, experience all there was to experience and not feel the least bit of regret for not doing what she wanted. At the same time, she didn't want to regret having done what she wanted because it in the end was not the right thing to do.

From: Lori Solomon6697@yahoo.com
'tis the day after …
shall we do that again from time to time?

From: Nick Warren557@hotmail.com
sounds maybe like a plan

Nick's last message was just enough to satiate the hunger of the wailing uncertainty that resided deep within her. After all, it was the day after, the traditional gray zone, where light met darkness, fire met frost, and delusion met reality. "Sounds maybe like a plan" spoke volumes to the little Pollyanna that occasionally jumped in place behind the Captain's wheel in Lori's head. "Sounds maybe like a plan" told her to keep steering the Queen of Mayhem, to keep moving forward despite the fact that there was no destination.

Two weeks passed. The all-business cyber messages she sent to Nick, regarding trivial radio-related matters that served mostly as transparent excuses for her to connect with him, apparently disintegrated in transit. She received no replies. She had only butterflies filling her stomach with unsettling vibration and ceaseless motion, horseflies filling her head with unyielding turmoil.

From: LoriSolomon6697@yahoo.com
why are you so into playing GAMES?

From: Nick Warren557@hotmail.com
what you mean girl?

From: LoriSolomon6697@yahoo.com
i send e-mails, you don't respond
why??

From: Nick Warren557@hotmail.com
ive just been busy with the billings

havent replied to any one … sorry hun

Lori supposed in her crazed, emotionally debilitated state she had little choice but to accept that. After all, the stale breadcrumb that had been thrown to the beggar was still edible; the bone tossed to the salivating dog still had some meat on it. She preoccupied herself just enough with school-related matters to give her some distance from the asphyxiating black hole of cyberspace for a full day and a half. Yet just because she was not physically banging away at a keyboard did not mean she didn't every half hour or so look over at the computer terminal and sigh wistfully into her textbooks.

From: LoriSolomon6697@yahoo.com
so are you planning on responding?

From: Nick Warren557@hotmail.com
hey i sent one yesterday i think i'm not sure …
our cart ready system died so ive been busy working on that and other technical junk

From: LoriSolomon6697@yahoo.com
i miss discussing … certain … things …
do you?

From: Nick Warren557@hotmail.com
say that again

From: LoriSolomon6697@yahoo.com
say what again?

From: Nick Warren557@hotmail.com
what you were wrote me earlier

From: LoriSolomon6697@yahoo.com
huh? what i was wrote you earlier?
translation?

From: Nick Warren557@hotmail.com
oh im sorry … just going nuts over here … hehe

     He was preoccupied. She wished that she, too, were preoccupied with something, anything other than him. The piercing pain of missing someone, of wanting to hear a voice, touch a hand, laugh at a misspelled word on a computer screen, was an agony she had grown to know too well in the time that she had known him.

From: LoriSolomon6697@yahoo.com
so do you miss talking about … things with me?

From: Nick Warren557@hotmail.com
ive just been busy hun. yeah i think about it

From: LoriSolomon6697@yahoo.com
think about … what exactly?

From: Nick Warren557@hotmail.com
things

From: LoriSolomon6697@yahoo.com
good things, or bad?

From: Nick Warren557@hotmail.com
i dunno

     I dunno. I dunno. What did that mean? Where was he coming from? What was on his mind? And how could Lori be so intrigued with someone past the age of twelve who used the phrase "I dunno?"

She allowed two days of excruciating anguish to unfold, two days of her overwhelming fixation to rattle and shake, and very nearly break her. For it was two full days of simply not knowing, yet fully understanding that the passing silence could easily be the most telling and hurtful of all.

From: LoriSolomon6697@yahoo.com
so what's your answer?
good thoughts, or bad?

From: Nick Warren557@hotmail.com
oops I deleted the email you were talking about after i read it
hehe. nah ive been pretty good lately. busy as hell. trying to work on a couple girls ive been flirting with on line. i got a date with one tomorrow night. Whoohooo.... yummy ... lol....

From: LoriSolomon6697@yahoo.com
so what does that mean?
do you still want to play, Nick?

From: Nick Warren557@hotmail.com
i'll be in the mood to play more

From: LoriSolomon6697@yahoo.com
we're still "playmates?"

From: Nick Warren557@hotmail.com
yeah

Lori didn't interpret his stinging candidness as a conscious attempt to hurt her. She might have if they were playing by traditional rules guided by normal, human expectations and intention. Yet they were doing anything but that.

Their periodic unions were like cream in coffee: there for taste, there for consumption, and swallowed in thirsty gulps by the passing night and the emerging dawn. There was no permanence, and certainly no commitment. A small part of her actually appreciated his unfiltered honesty; a small part of her believed it helped to define who they were to each other. Yet every so often, this same small part of her would allow itself to feel the empty sadness of impending loss, and fear and anxiety would rush in and replace her seeming indifference. Her personal bipolar cycle ran its own nauseating course while Nick's did the same. Unfortunately, their cycles rarely, if ever, seemed to coincide.

From: AngelontheAirwaves3254@hotmail.com
Subject: Re:
To: LoriSolomon6697@yahoo.com
I'd love to have din-din with you tonight. I hope you get this e-mail. Wanna meet at our usual place? PLEEEEEEEASE.... I NEEEEEEEEEEED TO SEEEEEEEEEEE YOU, MY LL/SF.
I'm actually growing my hair out another four to five inches. I can't wait for you to see how much longer it's gotten. I've been told that I look GREAT and very sexy with longer hair. That isn't to say, though, girlfriend, that one still doesn't need a good trim and shaping. Your hair looked a little frayed at the ends the last time I saw you. JUST a suggestion, LL/SF.
Angela

From: LoriSolomon6697@yahoo.com
Subject: Re:

To: AngelontheAirwaves3254@hotmail.com
I need to shower first. I've been going straight since five AM. Didn't have the chance to shower today.
Lori

From: AngelontheAirwaves3254@hotmail.com
Subject: Re:
To: LoriSolomon6697@yahoo.com
You disgusting floozy. Maybe you shouldn't shower. I kind of like the "sweaty, greasy" look. LOL!
Oh, lord! I have to appear on TV tomorrow. We're joining with Channel 7 in an all day telethon, and all the "talent" has to go on TV for an hour to beg for pledges. Yuck. I am WAY too fat for TV nowadays, and I am going to be SO self-conscious!!!!!!!!!!!!!!!!!!!!!!!!!!!!
Angela

From: LoriSolomon6697@yahoo.com
Subject: Re:
To: AngelontheAirwaves3254@hotmail.com
Oh, stop! You'll be great. Just focus on the higher purpose of your television appearance!

From: AngelontheAirwaves3254@hotmail.com
Subject: Re:
To: LoriSolomon6697@yahoo.com
screw the higher purpose.

From: LoriSolomon6697@yahoo.com
Subject: Re:
To: AngelontheAirwaves3254@hotmail.com
tramp

From: AngelontheAirwaves3254@hotmail.com
Subject: Re:
To: LoriSolomon6697@yahoo.com

you suck suck suck

From: LoriSolomon6697@yahoo.com
Subject: Re:
To: AngelontheAirwaves3254@hotmail.com
at least i don't randomly screw higher purposes
tart

From: LoriSolomon6697@yahoo.com
Subject: Re:
To: AngelontheAirwaves3254@hotmail.com
WHERE DID YOU GO???!!!!!!!!!!

From: AngelontheAirwaves3254@hotmail.com
Subject: Re:
To: LoriSolomon6697@yahoo.com
I'm here, I'm here. You can't keep me out late tonight,
because this telethon is going right into the evening and
I'm going to have to cover it as a news story in addition
to participating in it. Tomorrow is just going to be crazy.
And I'm already exhausted... Beyond exhausted. I'll tell
you about that later.

From: LoriSolomon6697@yahoo.com
Subject: Re:
To: AngelontheAirwaves3254@hotmail.com
I won't keep you out late. Promise.

From: AngelontheAirwaves3254@hotmail.com
Subject: Re:
To: LoriSolomon6697@yahoo.com
you'd better not, you little person who sucks!

When they arrived at the restaurant, Lori didn't
observe anything out of the ordinary with Angela's
appearance until they were sitting for a while at a table,

facing one another. Lori began to notice little dark folds of flesh under Angela's eyes. After they were served, she noticed Angela blinking hard while staring down at the slice of pizza in front of her. She slowly stripped slices of onions off of it and lethargically set them back on the surface of the remainder of the pie.

"We could have ordered it without, you know," Lori said.

"Lori, I barely know I'm alive. I'm too far-gone tonight to catch something like onions on pizza. I was up all night fretting about a million silly things."

"What kinds of silly things?" Lori asked, biting into her pizza, onions and all.

"Look at this," Angela said. She pushed against the tip of her nose with her forefinger. "Look how wide and visible my nostrils are. My nose turns up too much. When I first had it done, the job just wasn't done the right way. I'm thinking about having it done again, if they can."

"I like your nose. It gives your face character," Lori said.

Angela laughed. "I knew you'd say that. I knew you'd say 'character.' But everyone who knows me tells me that my nose isn't the right fit for my face. I hear this from *everyone*."

"Well, I think your nose is fine. But if it bothers you, then I'm all for doing something about it."

"Also I'm fat," Angela said. She lifted a lace-lined square of fabric dangling over the top half of the dress she was wearing. "I'm disgusting," she said, pointing to her abdomen.

"You're not disgusting, Angela. Come on. You're always way too hard on yourself."

"Look," Angela said. She stood up and turned sideways. "Look at this. *Look* at this!" She ran her hand across her stomach, trying hard to highlight for Lori its convex shape. She poked at it a few times with her finger so Lori could appreciate its thickness, density, and fluidity.

Lori sat in silence, not knowing what to say.

"I feel ugly and gross," Angela said.

"Angela, come on. You're very *attractive*. You dress beautifully. Your hair and make-up always look great. I mean," Lori paused. "Should you lose weight for health reasons? Y-yeeaah. It's your life, for Christ's sake, and I've told you this I don't know how many times. But I'm not gonna sit here and agree with you that you're gross or ugly. Because it's simply not true."

"Well, then, I have to disagree with *you* on not agreeing with *me*." She took a large sip of Cabernet Savignon. She set her glass down, and then lifted it back up to empty what was left in one gulp. "Look," she said, shaking her head. "I have to tell you that one other thing that was keeping me awake last night was *you*."

"Me?"

"You." Angela lowered her empty glass to the table and traced the rim of it with her pinky.

"What about me?" Lori asked, a string of pizza cheese dangling from her chin.

"Lori, I think that as long as you keep *any* kind of contact going with Nick, you're doomed. I don't care how much you *think* you might be finally 'getting to know' him. He'll give you any little crumb if he thinks he can keep you among his little reservoir of 'playmates.' He wants nothing more from you but sex. Nothing, Lori."

Lori's eyes fell. "I know," she said, softly.

"You know that I used to be 'hooked' on my version of Nick," Angela said. "At the time, I had no one in my life, and he came along when I was vulnerable. Yet, once I realized that sex was all he wanted, I cut him loose. I gave him *one chance* to redeem himself.

But that was it. It hurt," she said. "It hurt like hell, not to get that connection that I wanted. But *you cannot squeeze blood from a stone*. And some people are stones, Lori. Nick is one of them."

Lori nodded, feeling like she had the floppy head of a rag doll getting shaken by an irate toddler.

"It's *only* draining your energy!" Angela yelled. "And for a girl with *so much going on already*, why do you need this guy? Why can't you just cut him loose, Lori? You know, I think you need to be asking yourself more questions about *why* in hell you are continuing this and less about what makes Nick tick. The issue isn't him. *It is you*. You've got an extremely unhealthy attachment to this so-called 'person'... and that's a reflection of *you*, not *him*. He's obviously perfectly fine with who he is. It's *you* that wants him to change... be 'nicer,' more able to 'connect' emotionally. What is the "sickness" in *you* that seems hell-bent on getting that stone to bleed? Don't you see? He is a *sex machine*. He wants only sex from whomever he can get it, wherever, whenever. *Just drop him Lori*. Like a piece of bad, smelly rubbish. Your connection with him only brings you down to his level. Makes you seem just as scummy as he is. Which I know you aren't."

Lori dropped what was left of her pizza slice on her plate, figuring that this was a good time for her to lose her appetite. She slowly wiped the grease from her fingertips onto a napkin as she continued to listen to what Angela had to say.

"Look, Lori," she said, her tone softening. "I'm being this brutally honest with you because I love you. I love you so much ... partly because I see so much of myself in you. And I see that if you don't stop this craziness while you are ahead, you'll lose so much of what's really important to you. Please, Lori. I am begging you. Pleading with you … to get this poison *out* of your life. Forever. Never to look back."

Lori felt a tapping on her shoulder. A lean, black teenager with large, soulful eyes leaned his head in toward hers and opened his mouth. He was heavily inebriated, and in between slurs and heavy streams of saliva slipping out of the corner of his mouth and down his chin, he managed to say, "I hope you don't mind me listenin' in on yo convuhsation… But misshh, I get the impression that you ah only *hearin'* what yo friend is sayin' to you. You ah not *listenin'*. That guy… It *is* a guy you're talking about, ain't tit? I mean, it?"

Angela smiled at him and nodded. "It's a *jerk* we're talking about," she said.

The drunken boy continued. "Yeah. That guy is a jerk-*off* . You *listen* to your friend. Don't just *hear* huh. She's a good, good person. She's a good, good friend."

After they paid the check and walked out of the restaurant, Angela said, laughing, "That kid and I were making eye contact the whole time I was talking. I couldn't believe he started talking to us!"

"Angela," Lori said, putting her arm around her and leaning in closely. "The next time you see someone eavesdropping on our *private* conversation in the middle of a crowded restaurant, behind my turned back, could you please give me the heads up so my life's story isn't spilled out to someone who's so centrally and peripherally anesthetized with alcohol that they can't *swallow*?"

"But Lori," Angela said. "I'm taking his presence tonight to mean much more than you are. He made so much sense with what he said that I honestly think he's your guardian angel!"

As Lori hugged her good-bye, she said, "Figures that my guardian angel is a rip roaring drunk."

Chapter 20

*Grief is the agony of an instant, the indulgence of grief
the blunder of a life*
Benjamin Disraeli (1804-1881)

From: AngelontheAirwaves3254@hotmail.com
Subject: Re:
To: LoriSolomon6697@yahoo.com
LL/SF,
I just want to tell you that I REALLY appreciate the way you always "stick up" for me when I am complaining about either my weight or my nose. That is the sign of a really great friend, one who will accept me just the way I am.
I want you to understand that I am not just "dumping" on myself indiscriminately about everything. I want you to understand that I DO recognize all of my good points, as well as my bad. I've had a lot of work done on parts of my face- like having big circles under my eyes sucked out, wearing braces, and getting my teeth whitened when they'd become dull. But I NEVER went to extremes, like getting higher cheekbones, collagen in my lips, and so forth and so on. I realize that even with a better nose, my face won't ever be perfect (no one's is really, not even supermodels because they're all air-brushed). But you won't see me going to a plastic surgeon every other month for some other "procedure."
I just want you to know that the things that have bothered me over the years really SHOULD have bothered me. They were things that others noticed and suggested I get "fixed" so as to improve my looks. And they were not all that difficult TO fix, know what I mean? Sure, it was not fun to wear braces for five years (at two different times, to fix crooked bottom teeth and a big overbite). Nor was it fun to have the liposuction. But it

was WELL WORTH IT for the results. And once I lose the weight I want to lose, if I still have a paunch belly, I will consider having a tummy tuck. Sometimes, not even a thousand sit-ups a day will correct a potbelly. But that's probably the only other plastic surgery I would consider having. Except for a facelift in 20 or 30 years- if I need it. I really am lucky to have such great skin. That's one thing you will never hear me complain about. I think it is important that we accept ourselves as we are for the most part. I do think people "go under the knife" way too often and for too many things. But at the same time, there is also room for improvement in everyone. And in many cases, it is in our best interest to try to improve upon certain things. Do you understand what I'm saying?

I feel the exact same way about my personal and professional self. I want to continue to work on myself in every possible way, so as to be the best person Angela Allen can be. I want to LOOK as best I can, I want my broadcast work to be the best it can, and I want to be as good, sensitive, and compassionate a person as possible.

I hope it helps you understand where I am coming from on all of this.

Angela

Lori sat on a couch in the university library reading a chapter on cloning. As her eyes skimmed diagrams showing elaborate nucleotide sequences being elegantly spliced by "restriction enzymes" and magically glued back together by "ligases," she wondered how Nick was spending his Saturday evening. She wondered if Nick was wondering how *she* was spending her Saturday evening. She wondered if Nick was wondering why she was not spending it with him. She

231

wondered if Nick was wondering anything about her at all.

Genetic manipulation. Manipulation. All of Lori's thoughts seemed to melt into one as she pressed her back more deeply against the middle cushion of the couch and randomly flipped the pages of her textbook. It was not a night when she wanted to be studying. It was not a night when she wanted to be alone.

She headed home just as the darkened skies had begun to crack open with the insults of blinding lightning bolts. Cold streams of water pierced her skin the second she left her car and darted across the flooded parking lot to her apartment building. She lifted her drenched hand to her face and tried to wipe away the mucus that had just begun to drip from her nostrils, yet the gesture served only to cover cheeks and chin with discomforting wetness.

Once inside, she peeled off water saturated jeans and a sodden sweatshirt, and slipped into warm, dry jogging pants and a black concert t-shirt. She tried calling Paul. She waited with the phone resting between her chin and her shoulder as his phone rang and rang. Only the torpedoing of water pellets against the windowpane above her head stole from the emptiness of his absence on the other end of the line.

She leaned back against a pillow and held the phone against her chest. An hour passed before she sat upright on the twisted sheets strangling her bare mattress and realized that her thumb was starting to ache from pressing down on the receiver. The storm outside had picked up in intensity, hurling gusts of angry, heavy air against her bedroom window. The night sky turned bone white every so often, followed by flashes of cloudy darkness and earth-shaking explosions.

She could not get her mind off of Nick.

She moved lethargically over to the computer, rested her hands on the cedar wood table it sat on and bowed her head in front of it. She was dizzy from not having eaten anything for hours, yet she was feeling too weak and saddened to fill her stomach. She started to hack away at the keys of the computer in an attempt to escape into her writing.

She was so lonely.

She checked her e-mail, and saw that she had two messages. One was from Rutherford. The other was from Angela.

From: SeriousSchmendrick4428@aol.com
Subject: The Tao of my Balls
To: LoriSolomon6697@yahoo.com

I'm in a strange mood. On the one hand I'm content, but on the other, restless and suspicious. I'm eating vermicelli out of a stainless steel bowl and drinking water right out of the gallon-jug that it came in.

I spoke with Babette on the phone for about 2 hours last night. We had a good talk. She might even come here to visit next month. Ugh! Is this a *good* idea? I don't know! Dearest, you have no idea how complicated it is to be a male. I'm hearing "no, no, no!" from above the neck, but "yes, yes, yes!" from below the neck. It's a quandary, I tell you! Where is the middle ground? Being a "male" means being in a constant and irrepressible struggle between the brain and the weenie… and unfortunately, the weenie usually wins. No matter what the implications are, dammit, I still can't figure out why women don't rule the world! You've got the power! Men are so easy to manipulate! What's WRONG with you women?!

Respectfully submitted,

Rutherford (a.k.a. Philip Le C'est Bon)

From: AngelontheAirwaves3254@hotmail.com
Subject: Re:
To: LoriSolomon6697@yahoo.com

Lori,

I just wanted to share with you what happened at the doctor's office this morning. I weighed in at exactly 200 pounds. My doctor was FURIOUS with me. She said I need to lose an absolute minimum of 30 pounds, an average of 50, and eventually 70. She also switched my medication to one that will help curb my appetite in addition to speed up my metabolism. So, there you have it, right from the ol' doctor. I told her that some of my friends actually think I look good at my current weight. To which she gave me a smirky look and said, "You have to wonder what their motives would be, Angela. Are those so-called friends trying to give you excuses for staying at your current weight so that they can be sure they'll always look better than you? I am here to tell you that you do NOT look good. You look well over the standards for obesity, and I want you to be 30 pounds lighter the next time you enter my office. Or I will insist that you get into a 12-step program for an eating disorder."

Okay, Lori. That is a direct quote, and I NEEDED you to hear it. Having told you that, I must make it clear that I do NOT think for one minute YOU have been telling me I look good at my current weight so that you can feel somehow superior. But, I must admit, at times I have been truly perplexed as to why you would be the SOLE person in my world (including family, friends, even casual acquaintances) who ever tells me I look good at 180-200 pounds. It just has not made sense to me. So I have to ask you to please not EVER say that again, because it feels like an untruth from a very good friend, regardless of whether you mean it or not. And, more importantly, it has a VERY BAD effect on me; in my subconscious mind, it is literally enabling me NOT to take better care of myself. I am grossly overweight. That is the plain and simple truth, right from my doctor's mouth.

I respect the fact that you honestly think I don't look bad at my current weight. But please respect the fact that I am admitting that I have a big problem with food, and it has affected my appearance and my health. And I NEED HELP COMBATING IT. THAT DOES NOT LEAVE ANY ROOM FOR ME TO BE TOLD I LOOK GOOD.

I don't know how much clearer I can be about my needs on this issue.

Forgive me for coming on strong. It's very tough to finally come out of denial about a problem I've had for the last three years. This is serious business. It is NOT about having a few extra pounds. It has become a serious health issue for me, and quite frankly, it has scared the PISS out of me.

Angela

Lori felt her heart thumping hard in her chest. Her mouth was dry and her head was light, and she knew without looking in a mirror that some color had drained from her face. She hit the reply cue above Angela's message and started to type fast.

From: LoriSolomon6697@yahoo.com
Subject: Re:
To: AngelontheAirwaves3254@hotmail.com
Angela,
The clothes you were wearing the other night were very flattering, and this is true of the clothes you usually wear whenever I see you. It wasn't until you started lifting up flaps and pointing to trouble zones that I couldn't help but take notice of your weight gain.

When you've told me in the past what you weigh, and that your weight puts you at risk of having a heart attack or a stroke, have I ever ONCE told you that I thought it was healthy for you to carry so much weight around? I remember telling you the exact opposite countless times. And even then, did I ever really tell you something that you didn't already know? What could I possibly say to you that you can't see for yourself when you look in the mirror in the mornings or when you step on a scale in a doctor's office? I guess I just don't understand why you lean so heavily on others to reinforce what I see as already being obvious.

I feel that I've only ever tried to be a good friend to you. If you have friends that seriously want to keep you "down," that's really unfortunate, and I feel sorry that you have people like that in your life. As for me, I can't try any harder than I have been for so long to try to make you feel good, and to try to offer you advice that I think will make your life better. If you can't see that, then it's a problem you have with me that I can't do anything about.

Lori

Lori sighed and shut off her computer. She moved back toward her bed, leaned against the same upright pillow, and tried reading a novel that she had bought months earlier at a yard sale. Her eyes captured the words printed on the pages, yet nothing was penetrating.

She placed the book down on her comforter and drifted into her living room to see what was on television. After she passed all of the channels three consecutive times without seeing anything that she felt could hold her interest, she turned the power off and migrated back into her bedroom. The emerald green numbers on her clock shifted from 9:15 to 9:16 pm, and the sliding sound they made went rhythmically in sync with the rumbling of thunder and the tapping of rain droplets on her cold, foggy bedroom window.

The phone rang.

"Lesbian lover?" Angela said, meekly.

"Hi."

"I got your e-mail."

"Yes?"

"Look, Lori. I don't have a problem with you. I love you, and I *know* that you love me. And you really *have* been a great friend to me. Okay?"

"Okay..."

"*I'm the screwed up one here, okay*? I have an eating disorder and I have to come to terms with that. I'm angry. I'm hurt. I'm depressed, and I'm frustrated." She started to cry.

"Angela..." Lori started.

"I'm sorry if I seem to have taken all this out on you," she said, sobbing.

"It's okay," Lori said. "It's all right."

"It's... hard to explain how I feel, Lori." Angela muffled the receiver with her hand and blew her nose. "I do know that I feel like I just want to go to sleep and never wake up. I hate myself."

"Angela..."

"No. I hate my life. I hate everything." She continued sobbing.

"Come on, Angela," Lori said. "Are you going to be all right?"

"I'll be all right. I'll be all right." She blew her nose again. "I'm just having a really tough time right now."

"I know you are," Lori said.

"You always pull through for me, Lori, and I honestly don't know what I'd do without you. I'm so scattered and moody a lot of the time, and sometimes I don't feel like I'm being a good enough friend to you. I get so caught up in my own self-pity crap."

"Look, we all get moody. I know your heart's in the right place with me, and honestly, sometimes I don't see things clearly either. I'll always consider you to be a good friend. So *stop*."

"I think I'm in love with you." Angela giggled.

"Love you, too." Lori gently hung up the phone. She stared down at it for a few seconds before picking up the receiver and dialing Rutherford's number. She leaned her head back against a pillow.

"Hello?" a deep, solemn-sounding voice answered.

"Hi. It's me," Lori said. "Just read your latest e-mail."

"Lori!" Rutherford chirped. "It's been a while. I mean, since we've actually *spoken* to one another."

"Yes it has," Lori said. "How are you?" she asked.

"I'm broke," he said. "All I've got is this cat that sits on the other side of my room and occasionally falls into my toilet. Come over here, Boo Bear." He shuffled the phone. "Not right on papa's groin. On papa's thigh. There. Lori. It was the funniest thing. All of a sudden... plunk! I had to wash the blue crap off her." He took a gulp of something before saying, "Could you just wait a second? I have to pee very badly."

Lori waited with the phone resting between her chin and her shoulder. She heard him shut a door in the distance.

"I'm back," Rutherford breathed into the phone.

"So... I started finally doing little science updates for radio," Lori said.

"Really? Hey, hey. Congratulations."

"They're not airing too many, but I'm patient."

"You know what?" he said. "I helped make this jingle that they still play here on some of the local stations." He cleared his throat and started singing in a soft, high voice, "Everybody loves Jack Burns... Everybody loves Jack Burns... Everybody, everybody, everybody, everyboooody... Everybody loves Jack Burns!"

"Huh... Did you now?" Lori asked. "That's pretty cool. You wrote it, and came up with the tune?"

"No. Someone else did that. I just convinced them to change the guy's name from Dick." He started laughing uproariously into the receiver.

Lori leaned back and let Rutherford fill her ears with tales of sickness, torture, injustice, and Babette. An hour passed. She waited for an appropriate break in Rutherford's monologue so she could segue off the phone.

She was still restless. She thumbed her little black "at a glance" address book and scanned the pages for more potential distractions. When her eyes fell on Nick Warren's cell phone number, she hesitated for a few seconds. She quickly dialed it, not bothering to enter star 67 this time to veil her identity. The phone rang and rang.

He was not there. Or, more than likely he was there, studying her number on his caller I.D., and just not answering. Lori slowly hung up the phone. Her stomach twisted into a taut braid. She listened to the sound of raindrops, and nervously played with a callous on the upper side of her palm. She walked over to her computer and logged into her e-mail account.

From: AngelontheAirwaves3254@hotmail.com
Subject: Re:
To: LoriSolomon6697@yahoo.com
I came away from that conversation feeling so very good. It's undeniable how much we both love and care

for one another. This friendship is very important to the both of us. I love you so very much, Lori. You are a one-of-a-kind friend... and I NEVER want to lose you.

We have a "clean slate" now... and there is no reason to ever have another nasty episode again. Don't you agree?

So... are we back to being LL/SF again??? I sure hope so!!!!!

Angela

Lori logged out. She pushed her chair away from her desk and threw herself onto her bed. She lay down on her stomach, clutching her chin with her fist. She fluttered her legs and felt the muscles in her calves tense. Thoughts of Paul began to form a pale haze in her head, a distorted image, worn and faint from time that had passed since she last saw him. She wished at that moment that he was by her side, telling her how much he loved her, how much she meant to him, how she had changed his life by choosing to be with him. But instead she had chosen to be on her own. She had chosen to be so miserably on her own.

Her stomach felt achy and empty, yet she was anything but hungry. She picked at the dry skin on her hand and flicked a flake over the side of her bed. The allure of Nick Warren seemed ridiculous to her, his once-shimmering image dull and lifeless in light of the stinging reality that … she was alone. She moved to the edge of her bed. She began to reach for the phone receiver, pulling herself away only at the realization that there was no one to talk to.

She needed Nick to know that she did not need him. She did not need his touch. She did not need his validation. She did not need his control. But she did need for him to know that she *did not need him*. She called his cellular phone, not protecting her identity by pushing any codes because she wanted him to be aware of whom it was trying to get in touch with him. She listened to his voice-mail. She lowered the receiver and redialed. She listened to his voice-mail again. She left him a message asking him to call her back.

He never did.

The following morning, she called him at work, figuring that she had probably scared him off by not making any references to screwing in her recorded message.

"WBUZ..." a black woman's voice rang out.

"Hello," Lori said. She assumed one of the receptionists had answered. "Is Nick Warren there?"

"Uh ..." She paused for a moment. Lori thought she could hear his distinctly nasal, New England-accented voice in the distance. "Heeeeeee's ... uh ... he's away from his ... desk right now."

"Oh," Lori said. "Should I hang on?"

"Well ..." The woman sounded distracted, and must have placed her palm over the receiver for a few seconds because Lori suddenly couldn't hear anything. "Why don't you ... leave a message on his voice-mail?"

"Um ... I'll call back later. Thanks."

"O-kay," she said. The woman's voice sounded strained.

Did the little blue or green man inside Lori's head detect suppressed laughter? Was this woman screening his calls? Did she know who Lori was? Did Nick tell her who she was? Did he tell anyone who she was? Why *didn't* he return her call?

Her face started to feel warm, and the skin on the back of her neck began to tingle. She gathered her coat and her purse and hastily decided that she needed to face down the truth, even if the truth was manifested as her most neurotic prophecy. She walked quickly and purposefully to her car, envisioning everyone at the radio station crowding around his desk and gazing in disbelief at the screen of his computer.

"Yeah, so she sent me these," she pictured him boasting to his colleagues. "Get a load of this one!"

"She wrote *that*?"

"*Lori*? *Lori* wrote that? To … *you*?"

Laughter. Gasps.

"I don't believe it!"

Amazed silence.

"Yeah." She could see him shrugging helplessly. "And now she's callin' me at home. She's callin' me here at work. I can't get rid of her! Thanks, Shelly, for mannin' my phone."

"You poor thing, you." Lori could picture Shelly, the garish, black receptionist, patting his back and shaking her head and smirking.

Lori arrived at the station. As she passed through the narrow hallway leading to the office cubicles, she anticipated the worst. She saw arms reaching out to restrain her while she violently threw shadow punches at Nick, and she saw her already precarious position as science reporter at the station die an embarrassing, instantaneous death.

To her relief, upon rounding the corner of the corridor, what greeted her was not a band of leering, suspicious eyes, skulking, cowering silhouettes, and chilly silence, but rather the heartwarming pandemonium of a radio station's midday administrative and production staff.

"Hi, Lori!" Bob, one of the producers yelled out. He shuffled a stack of paper and smiled broadly at her before sitting down at his desk.

"Hey, Lori!" Sharon Warsaw, the station's lead news reporter called to her with a long strand of sour kraut dangling from the corner of her grinning mouth.

"Pardon me," she said, with a laugh, shoving it quickly between her greasy lips.

"Lori! How are your studies going?" an engineer named Chet asked as he made his way to a nearby water cooler.

"Fine," she responded. She felt her hands quivering beneath the pockets of her button-down sweater.

She saw Jonathan standing in back of the desk in his office, leaning over it to kiss his wife lightly on the lips. His wife smiled at him and caressed his cheek before heading off to his upstairs financial advising firm with a stack of papers pressed against her chest. They seemed so normal. They seemed so happy. Lori wondered if she, herself, would ever know of such normality and such happiness.

"Hey, there," she heard Nick say in a high-pitched voice as Lori neared his desk. "What brings you here?"

"I--"

"Hey," he interrupted. "I'm sorry I didn't get back to you the other day." He stared at the screen of his computer and began typing something. "I wasn't feelin' well. Had to go in for a biopsy yesterday and they loaded me up with narcotics. Passed out around six-thirty or seven last night."

She glanced over to the center of his desk, where a large solitary rose sat in a tall glass vase, looming over a stack of CDs and minidisks. Because he never talked about it, she still found herself often forgetting about the transplant. She'd frequently forget that he was walking around with someone else's heart. The heart of someone she'd never know.

"Can we talk?" she asked.

"Sure," he said. "What about?"

She looked up briefly at the others, who were talking amongst themselves. "Can we go... around the corner to talk? Away from everyone?"

"No," he said cheerily, with raised eyebrows. "Let's just talk here."

"Come on," she said. "Let's go somewhere else."

"I'm not budging."

"Why not?" she asked.

His eyebrows sunk deeply in his forehead, and his voice became very low. "Because it will look *bad*."

Any fears Lori had of Nick betraying her trust disappeared. The blasé attitude of his peers and his steadfast reluctance to be seen even walking around a corner with her told her everything she needed to know. She bowed her head, leaned closer to him, and bent her body partly over the counter lining one side of his desk. "O.K.," she whispered, careful to talk only when the hum of voices in the background was loud enough to drown her out. "I've been doing some thinking. No more e-mails. No more phone calls."

"I don't want to talk about this here," he said quietly, sternly.

"You're not leaving me with any choice, are you?" she said.

He glanced quickly up at her, and then directed his eyes at his computer screen, making sure to keep his fingers dancing busily against the keyboard as she continued.

"Things are too up and down with you," she said. "There's all this intensity, then there's nothing."

"But that's me," he interjected. "That's the way I am."

"But that's not the way I am," she said.

"But that's me. That's the way I am," he repeated, as if programmed like the computer in front of him.

"Look at me," she said.

He peered up at her face.

"That's not the way *I* am," she said, slowly and methodically. "There are two of us here. It's not just you."

He just sat there, staring straight into her face with his cavernous, glacial blue eyes, giving off the impression that he was truly listening to what she was saying, perhaps even affected by it. Yet Lori had a feeling that she knew what he was really thinking.

Yeah. Oh, well.

He kept his eyes fixed intently on Lori's as she walked slowly away from his desk. He said nothing, but continued to stare at her with a blank expression.

The rose became a red blur in the corner of Lori's eye as she continued to distance herself from him. She could hear it whispering to her. Was it whispering? No. It was hissing at her, trying desperately to make her understand that Nick was living his life in a way that was different from most. His fears were buried in an attempt to try to get as much out of life as he could in the short amount of time he was told that he had. Emotional attachments and all the stresses and annoyances that went with them could only get in the way of Nick living his life the way *he* wanted to live it. His mortality was fueling him, and Lori was only standing in the way. The rose continued to sputter. She pictured its stem bending forward and all of its petals pointing in unison toward the corner of the wall from behind which Lori had disappeared. If she could just open her eyes and unmire herself from the sloppy mess of her own demons, maybe she could finally see what the hell was going on.

Chapter 21

Think with the wise but walk with the vulgar
German Proverb

From: SeriousSchmendrick4428@aol.com
Subject: Do ants eat pee?
To: LoriSolomon6697@yahoo.com
Dear Lori,
Babette's clinging to our little "thing," and I just don't have the heart to tell her that we're at the end of the road. The problem is, Lori, that I want it BOTH ways, you know? I don't want to totally be rid of her, because I do like traveling out to see her occasionally, but it's not fair to anybody to continue like this. Right now all I've been doing is blowing it off and discouraging her from coming here, and even though she invited me out there I keep coming up with excuses why I can't do it. I guess neither one of us just wants to say "seeya!" like we should. All I know is that I'm sick of the whole thing, and believe it or not I do feel guilty about wanting to get involved with other people while she's out there thinking that there is some chance we'll eventually be together or something. I'm tired of these goofy "relationships" I've been having … married women, dysfunctional psychos, McDonalds drive-thru cashiers … You name it. All I want is a girl who is around my own age, has a sense of humor, lets me play Pac Man until three AM, and isn't afraid to slap me in the head and tell me to get a life. Is that too much to ask?! She doesn't have to be a Swedish aerobics instructor, for Christ's sake, although I could probably be persuaded to quit playing Pac Man should one come along.
Rutherford

From: LoriSolomon6697@yahoo.com

Subject: Re:
To: SeriousSchmendrick4428@aol.com
I keep thinking about Nick.
Lori

From: SeriousSchmendrick4428@aol.com
Subject: Wishful thinkin'
To: LoriSolomon6697@yahoo.com
Lori, if I live to be a hundred years old, I'll never figure out what your deal is with this guy. Nick just wants to get laid, Lori. Do you understand? I guarantee you that he laughs at you behind your back and probably tells all of his friends what a ditz you are. Believe me, I know. Stop wasting your time thinking about that idiot. Mark me words. I know you won't listen, but you need to just ignore that guy. Don't talk to him, don't look at him, don't answer or even OPEN his e-mails, hang-up on him if he calls you; do whatever you gotta do. ANY ENERGY WHATSOEVER that you contribute to this crap is only going to let him know that you still want him. Even if you walked up to him and spit in his face and kicked him in the crotch that would STILL be giving him attention and thus encouraging his advances. Trust me.
I'll talk more later.
OY VEY!
Rutherford

Ditz? Did he call her a ditz? Lori had taken some hard hits from Rutherford before, but never like this. She started writing her response to him, and then erased it. Then she started writing again. She drew a deep breath, let out a long sigh, and walked away from the computer for a few minutes to calm down.

From: LoriSolomon6697@yahoo.com

Subject: Re:
To: SeriousSchmendrick4428@aol.com
Is that what YOU do with all the girls you've had your way with? Laugh at them behind their backs, and giggle to all your friends about what ditzes they are??
Lori

From: SeriousSchmendrick4428@aol.com
Subject: Re: angry e-mail #1
To: LoriSolomon6697@yahoo.com
No. That's not what I do, but I know plenty of guys who do.

From: LoriSolomon6697@yahoo.com
Subject: Re:
To: SeriousSchmendrick4428@aol.com
I've been looking at you as this almost guru of the soul-less numbskulls out there… Trying so hard to get some insight. But you know? I think every situation is different. Every person is different. I may never be able to really understand why I've had what I've had with this guy, but I don't think I'm going to get anymore answers about it by looking to you for them.
Yes, I'm pissed. You hit a nerve.
I have enough guys in my life supposedly trying to "demean me" without needing you to make me feel like a complete moron.
Lori

From: SeriousSchmendrick4428@aol.com
Subject: Re: angry e-mail #2
To: LoriSolomon6697@yahoo.com
Every person and every situation is not necessarily that different, incidentally. There are patterns of human gender-specific behavior that are age-old and completely predictable. One of them is for people to get

highly defensive and angry when you tell them something they don't want to hear. I'd hope you'd respect the fact that I don't sit here and gloss-over anything. What do you expect me to say? "Gee, that Nick sounds like such a nice guy with good intentions?" Do you BELIEVE that? Think of it this way...if he really GAVE a crap about you, do you think he'd be making your life so difficult? Once again, I apologize if you feel that I've insulted your intelligence, but frankly I'm disturbed by how much energy you waste thinking about that knucklehead. If you think I'm WRONG about this, then do what you've gotta do and I'll keep my mouth shut from now on and we'll see what happens.

I'm certainly not trying to "demean" you in any way. I should have known that you'd get so angry eventually. In fact, when I sent that e-mail, I said, "uh-oh" right afterwards. I wasn't using my head, I admit, but that's not to say that I'm retracting the gist of what I said. I just wish I'd said it differently.

Oh, come on! Don't get so mad at me! You know I love you! I just word things in an insensitive way sometimes (or maybe all the time). You're my only real female confidante, and I don't want you to hate me or feel like you can't talk to me. Don't you realize that if two people of opposing genders can be totally HONEST with each other about their respective situations and perspectives that it might be a major breakthrough for all humanity? The two of us could be pioneers in the reconciliation of the male/female conflict, I hope.

Rutherford

From: LoriSolomon6697@yahoo.com
Subject: Re:
To: SeriousSchmendrick4428@aol.com
He's been a strange figment in my life that I just haven't been able to figure out what to do with. All I can say is

that by distancing myself from all of this for a little while, I'm hoping to get back on track.
Lori

From: SeriousSchmendrick4428@aol.com
Subject: Calling all dorks
To: LoriSolomon6697@yahoo.com
Okay. As a MALE, I know EXACTLY what that Nick clown is up to, and I find it absolutely stupefying that girls can get caught up in such horsecrap. I don't even need to MEET the guy, Lori. I know his whole game, and in fact, as you pointed out, I've played the same cards myself. The problem is, I certainly don't LIKE the fact that such a game is played, and when I see female friends of mine being manipulated I get this "father" complex or something and I want to grab you by the arms and shake you and scream "He's a DICK! He doesn't CARE about you! Wake UP!" I apologize for being judgmental. I just want you to be happy and free of internal conflict.
Anyway, I'll try *not* to be judgmental. It'll never work, of course, but I'll try. You aren't the first person to rip me for being arrogant and insensitive, but I swear to God I don't do it maliciously. It's only because I like you so much... really...
Until later, I remain...
Rutherford

From: LoriSolomon6697@yahoo.com
Subject: Re:
To: SeriousSchmendrick4428@aol.com
It still amazes me that guys will go to such lengths for a one-time thing. It just seems so empty and fruitless. I'd understand if the chase led to something more substantial, something with a little longevity and depth. But ... What's the point? I mean, if the relationship is

good, wouldn't the guy want a steady diet of it? I wish you, as a guy who has apparently done this in the past, would explain it to me. What's the allure? Surely there must have been SOME redeeming qualities in the girls that you were drawn to?

Does a guy with this type of mindset have the ability to care about a girl? Or is a womanizer completely clueless about connecting or communicating with a woman? What about loneliness?

I wish I could be a guy, with that kind of guy's brain, for just one day. Just one day. So I could understand.

Lori

From: SeriousSchmendrick4428@aol.com
Subject: Recalling all dorks
To: LoriSolomon6697@yahoo.com

A guy's "brain" is not what you need to understand us. You need to have a PENIS for a while. The brain and the penis are mutually exclusive entities. You have no idea how hard it is to have a penis (sorry, couldn't resist that one).

It's all a matter of biology and evolution, plain and simple and easy. Males of ALL species are genetically predisposed to release massive amounts of sperm in any direction possible to fertilize as many eggies as possible to keep the chain of life going. Females, on the other hand, only produce small amounts of eggies to be fertilized, and then there is a long period not only of gestation but of care for the offspring as well, so obviously it is in the female interest to look for something "with a little longevity," as you put it. That's IT. That explains all male and female behavior in my opinion, period. Of course, humans, unlike other species, DO have some rudimentary sense of morality, responsibility, loyalty, right, wrong, etc. etc., that tends to complicate our matters far more than what happens in the "brute" kingdom; but that will NEVER change our brute nature. You can't beat it. You can only hope to contain it.

I must go now. My friend Dan just showed up, and we're going to drink beer, get baked, eat some cheese and Mako Shark, and go "ugh! ugh! ugh!" and talk about how much we need to get laid.

Rutherford

Chapter 22

Life is half spent before we know what it is
George Herbert (1593-1633)

Lori was still plagued by a desire that she could not control. All she could do was try to will it away, like a dull ache in one's back muscles after sitting stationary in the same awkward position for too long. The less she focused on it, the less she figured it would bother her.

But it was still there.

From: SeriousSchmendrick4428@aol.com
Subject: Seize this ...
To: LoriSolomon6697@yahoo.com
I'm free next week for a potential lunchable interlude. I'm on a new diet, by the way. I'm tired of feeling like crap. I'm tired of looking down and seeing my gut instead of my prodigious manliness. I'm also tired of starting every sentence in this message with "I'm ..." That's kind of egotistical, don't you think?
Anyway, the next time we have lunch, don't let me order any fried clams or crap like that. I'll get the alfalfa burger, with a side order of hot water. I'd like to lose enough weight in the next few months so that I can feel comfortable mowing my lawn without a shirt on. There's nothing worse than a shirtless fat guy, wouldn't you agree? Lately I've felt so fat that I even wear my shirt in the shower. That way I can feel thinner and wash my shirt as the same time. The thing that sucks the most about having shaved my beard and gotten a haircut is that my lack of head-hair makes me look fatter. I look like a big fat dork with short hair and duplicity of chins right now. I don't like it. I've got to be the only clown in

the world with no chin who actually has two chins. A goatee may be in order.
Rutherford

The loud drumming of the Commuter Rail rocked the canals of Lori's ears as the train rapidly approached. She stepped into it, sat down in the nearest empty seat she could find, and began staring thoughtlessly out the window at the blackened, passing landscape. She stayed on the train as long as she was able to. She wanted to see nothing, to hear nothing, to feel nothing. She wanted to be in a complete void, a soothing, distancing, dulling state of sheer darkness. She wanted no light, no music, no poetry, and no conversation. She wanted to be so alone that it did not feel real, yet just real enough for her to embrace her own arms and rock herself gently in rhythm to the swaying movements of the train against the tracks.

As the train approached a stop, it slowed down in such a way as to propel all bodies on it forward. Lori had to bear her heels down hard on the floor to keep from being thrust into a neighboring seat. A wave of nausea forced her to close her eyes and rest her cold knuckles against her clammy forehead. Once the train pulled away from the platform and started to chug again evenly against the rails, she leaned her head against the cool metal wall next to her and began to feel some relief. The squeaking of the breaks grew fainter as the rocking motion of the train made her drift into a light slumber.

From: SeriousSchmendrick4428@aol.com
Subject: Chi-zeese and mac
To: LoriSolomon6697@yahoo.com
Dearest of the Dear,

Art cold? Why hast thou been silent? How now, sirrah!? Anon! Our great beacon has gone out? Hear more than thou knowest; set less than thou throwest. Leave thy drink and thy whore, and keep in a door, and thou shalt have more than two tens to a score.

What's up?

I need to hear your VOICE so that my increasing paranoia that you are actually a sinister FBI operative can be pacified. If you call here, ask for me as "Raskolnikov." Say, "Is Raskolnikov at home?" My secret agent KGB-defective name is "Rodion Romanovich Raskolnikov." The British know me as "Unya de Gato." The African nation knows me as "Johnny Fajita."

Yours in Bodhisattva,

Rutherford

At home again, Lori lay face down on her unmade bed, blowing her nose and dabbing her eyes with a tissue. She cried for a long time, pausing only to toss her used Kleenex into a bulging trash bag. She buried her face in her pillow and thought about holding her breath until she had reached the verge of blacking out. Then she thought about pressing the pillow tightly against her mouth and nose so that no air could get through. The thoughts passed. She quietly stood up, lifted the blankets off her bed, and shook them. She coughed as a cloud of dust rose and thickened the stale air.

From: SeriousSchmendrick4428@aol.com
Subject: her armpits
To: LoriSolomon6697@yahoo.com

Dearest,

I am not having ANY luck with my phone calls lately. I'm now 0-4 with you in the last 2 days. I don't know.

Cogito, ergo sum. Sin qua non. Dominus vobiscum et cum spiritu tuo. Unya de Gato vuelando como una paloma.

Let's do THIS... Just CALL me at exactly 6:30 pm on Friday evening. If you've got something else going on, let me know expediently, because if you DON'T call me I'll assume that my suspicions about you being a KGB operative are correct. Go back to Russia! You're a Soviet Kremlinite Cawmniss! What have you done with Lori?!

Rutherford

She sat outside her apartment on the top of a set of concrete steps. She closed her eyes, and taking long, deep breaths of the breezes swimming across her face she imagined a vast, pitch-black emptiness, much like the tunnel described by those close to death. She sat very still for a long while, with her eyes tightly shut and her head tilted back slightly. Apart from hearing an occasional car drive by, or the howling protests of a chained neighborhood dog, she felt consumed by what seemed to be an almost simulated pilgrimage to death. She was gliding away from the blinding, sour light of existence, falling through the beautiful passageway leading to eternal happiness...

From: SeriousSchmendrick4428@aol.com
Subject: Looooooooser
To: LoriSolomon6697@yahoo.com

Lori,

Everything just seems to suck, and I don't know why. It sounds cliché, but it's all so MEANINGLESS! The entire stratum of existence is like a pot of boiling water, and our lives are nothing more than fleeting little bubbles that rise to the top and pop into a steamy void. Oddly enough, I know exactly what the ANSWER is to everything, I think, but I just can't work out the dynamics of the equation involved, and therein lay an absence of reconciliation. I used to think I could divorce myself from any depressing ripples in the collective consciousness, but I'm sensing it all around me right now, and I'm both disturbed and intrigued by a growing sense of hopelessness that I don't think is unique to any single human being or even seemingly independent cultures.

I don't know what's up or down, and I'm not sure I even care.

Rutherford

Lori felt herself slipping away. She thought wistfully back to the time when she made sand castles with her brother, her parents sunning themselves nearby on a patch of beach with lotion on their noses and an umbrella over their heads. She could see it as if it were just yesterday. It was over a decade ago.

Life was over in a blink. Sex was over in a blink. There was impermanence to everything, even memories, which eventually also had a tendency to evaporate with time.

She couldn't help but think about Nick, and what life was like for him. Honestly. All considered. Day to day. Minute to minute. Second to second. Not knowing when would be the last batch of sunny-side up eggs and hashbrowns you'd ever have the chance to taste on a sun-drenched spring morning, or when would be the last hot, candle-lit bubble bath you'd ever have the pleasure of soaking in while reading a cheap, paperback novel. Not that anyone, no matter who they were or what their story, could ever really know, given the haphazard way life had a tendency to be. But it was still different with Nick. It was still very different, and it made Lori wonder.

The sky had gone from a rich auburn to a dark, dismal gray. Lori ambled slowly along a wide road flanked by sparse streetlamps and dark, expansive cornfields, a balmy wind blowing against her face as she closed in on a cluster of tombstones. She had to walk around an ornamental wrought iron fence to get near them, and to trail her hand across their rough, curvy surfaces. She paused only to skip over an occasional rock that had been placed on top of a few in memory of the resting loved one that lay beneath it.

It wasn't too long ago that they had buried her grandmother in that graveyard. She was lowered into one half of a double burial plot near Lori's grandfather. The two had always quarreled rancorously during the time Lori had known them, with squabbles culminating, at times, in fits of rage. Yet her grandmother's spirit passed on only a few months after her grandfather's body died. And now both would be by each other's side for eternity.

Lori knelt before the tombstone, and felt a soft wind pass over her and through the leaves on some nearby pine trees and blueberry bushes. She leaned back slightly and rested her palms against the cool earth behind her. A dust-filled gale made her eyes tear as it picked up debris and carried it across the graveyard. She pulled some scraggly weeds from the ground and matted down the uprooted soil with her fingertips.

Paul had been with her the day they buried her grandmother. He had held her tightly as they shoveled dirt back into the hole they had dug for her. As the biting cold wind of that day gusted and tousled their hair and tried nudging them from where they stood, Paul had continued to hold her tightly in his arms.

Restless, she walked over to a wind-tossed bouquet and picked it up. She dug a hole, small but deep, in front of the tombstone and crammed the stems into it. She patted the soil around the flowers and made them stand at a tilt in the dirt, and then turned and walked back to the open gate of the graveyard. A gentle wind hit her from behind and sent some of her hair flying forward. She turned to face the breeze, taking one long look at the cemetery before continuing back into the world of the living.

From: LoriSolomon6697@yahoo.com
nick,
do you want to resume what we had before?
just a "yes" or "no."
lori

From: NickWarren557@hotmail.com
yes

From: LoriSolomon6697@yahoo.com
i'd like very much to make you feel good again.
just let me know how, when and where

From: NickWarren557@hotmail.com
wow …
are you serious?
in which way are you talkin about

From: LoriSolomon6697@yahoo.com
the same way we're always talking about

From: NickWarren557@hotmail.com
tell me straight forward!
in which way
give me description

From: LoriSolomon6697@yahoo.com
tell me what you want

From: NickWarren557@hotmail.com
why now again?
i thought no more?

From: LoriSolomon6697@yahoo.com
i changed my mind

From: NickWarren557@hotmail.com
ahh i see….

From: LoriSolomon6697@yahoo.com
i just want to make you feel good
something about that makes me feel good

From: NickWarren557@hotmail.com
ahh ok …
what u gonna do with me when you see me
TELL ME IN DETAIL

The connection was re-established. She had capriciously reached out as one mere mortal to another, floundering aimlessly on this strange little planet with the constant threat of demise looming quietly and incessantly over their delicate porcelain heads. She craved his touch. She wanted his validation.

But could she handle his control?

She knew she wanted him, as part of the finite, miserable blur of her life. But suddenly and unexpectedly, she just wasn't sure to what extent. Fear of being hurt, fear of hurting, and fear of being consumed with poignant anxiety and confusion again were making her think and behave exactly as Nick had a tendency to behave toward *her*. And yet her passion toward him, her need to be bonded with him, made it impossible for her to loosen the grip she had so whimsically tightened around his loins.

Chapter 23

Good as drink is, it ends in thirst
Irish Proverb

From: NickWarren557@hotmail.com
so we meeting tonight?

From: LoriSolomon6697@yahoo.com
i really want to see you
but i think this week will be hard

From: NickWarren557@hotmail.com
well let's see … you want to see me … how about on
your way home tonight

From: LoriSolomon6697@yahoo.com
it's going to be late
sunday? i don't know

From: NickWarren557@hotmail.com
you really want it dont you …

The idea of having Nick so at bay was a decadent
thrill that, like a juicy page-turner of a mystery novel she
simply could not lay to rest. This ironic twist of power
lulled her into a delightful state of comfort and security
that she had not up to that point known with him. The
options to have or be had, to play or be played, danced
in synchronous harmony before her eyes like Can-Can
girls in a Las Vegas nightclub. It was all so clear now,
how Nick had been mischievously dealing the hands
this whole time. Except now it was she who was the
house, and the chips were most definitely stacked in
her favor.

From: LoriSolomon6697@yahoo.com
sorry i didn't respond
our server's been down since yesterday

From: NickWarren557@hotmail.com
SO TONIGHT OR ??

From: LoriSolomon6697@yahoo.com
i think i'll be studying until late tonight

From: NickWarren557@hotmail.com
so let's meet and eat and …

From: LoriSolomon6697@yahoo.com
next week, promise

A couple of days went by. She found herself hungering for a light snack. Nothing too filling. Just a nibble. A naughty little taste of more of Nick's forbidden fruit. She wondered how long she could succeed in having everything on her terms, just as Nick had managed to have with her for so long. She wondered exactly when the tides would turn, and when the power would be shifted to a different set of fortuitous hands. Perhaps she could find a way to keep the game going indefinitely, like leading a horse with a dangling carrot or sugar cane to the ends of the earth.

From: LoriSolomon6697@yahoo.com
do i have a chance for redemption?

From: NickWarren557@hotmail.com
anytime
what do think about tomorrow night

From: LoriSolomon6697@yahoo.com
yes

From: NickWarren557@hotmail.com
so tomorrow night we meet up and do it all!!!
what do you want to do?

From: LoriSolomon6697@yahoo.com
i want to make you feel good

From: NickWarren557@hotmail.com
so tomorrow night is it … where do you want to go?

From: LoriSolomon6697@yahoo.com
wherever the winds and the tides carry us

She did not hear from Nick until the following morning, an early bird still seemingly intent on catching the worm…

From: NickWarren557@hotmail.com
Hmm … the ack of my car?

From: LoriSolomon6697@yahoo.com
if we can find the "ack" of your car, then more power to us

From: NickWarren557@hotmail.com
i meant back of it.

She was thoroughly enjoying the flirtation, yet still ambivalent about seeing him in person. She used the busy day she had ahead of her as an excuse to cut their e-mail correspondence short. She decided to passively wait for him to reach out again to her, for if he wanted her as much as he seemed to, she would undoubtedly hear from him.

The evening came and went.

There were no phone calls.

There were no visits.

There was only an aura of mild curiosity circling around her as she drove home late the following evening from the library along the darkened, vacant highway. She felt no real disappointment, though, which only added to the already existing sense of command that she had been harboring for days. She knew that what had happened the previous night was the result of an unwritten standoff between her and Nick. He had been hoping to regain the power he realized he had lost, at least for now. What he didn't realize was that she wasn't about to give it back to him anytime soon. She was having far too much fun.

She initiated another flurry of e-mail messages the next day, a flurry of coolness on her end and coolness on Nick's end and no signs of breakthrough or resolution for either one of them. The battle of their respective egos had caused them both to lose an evening or two. Such a loss would have been devastating to her months or even weeks earlier, but for now it was just some annoyingly misplaced time. Because she knew deep down that this was all it was to Nick. Annoyingly misplaced time.

From: NickWarren557@hotmail.com
friday night?

From: LoriSolomon6697@yahoo.com
possibly, but you've got to *call* me! i do not possess a crystal ball!

From: NickWarren557@hotmail.com

well you know my cell number

From: LoriSolomon6697@yahoo.com
just let me know which night is best

From: NickWarren557@hotmail.com
friday night
i know you want mine bad

From: LoriSolomon6697@yahoo.com
and i know you want me

From: NickWarren557@hotmail.com
yes i do

   Friday night came, and Friday night went with a courtesy call from Lori explaining that she was too busy with her studies to make it happen. For the next several weeks, there were many nights like Friday night, interspersed between daily e-mail exchanges shamelessly and exhaustively expressing the most profound of each of their carnal desires. Generally, she found herself looking more forward to the promise of fantasy in their cyberspace exchanges than to the inevitable anticlimactic reality of their occasional unions. Yet even their e-mail correspondence was tainted by Nick's age-old tradition of turning up the heat and intensity to almost unbearably high levels, only to extinguish her with frosty silence on any given, random day.
   His world seemed meaningless to Lori, an endless circle of repetition with no real beginning and no definitive end. Whether it was the mysterious Mona seeking fleeting solace and refuge in the musty basement of his faceless papa, or Lori Solomon snapping painfully back like an elastic rubber band

wrapped around his thumb and forefinger, his world seemed to be very, very cyclical. And very, very empty.

It was Nick's tradition to whip into her life like a tornado, and cause confusion, folly, and mayhem. And only as the cloudy dust was just starting to settle back in its place, would Nick disappear like a child's hot breath swept up by a gentle breeze on a crisp autumn day.

Chapter 24

*Insanity: doing the same thing over and over again and
expecting different results*
Albert Einstein (1879-1955)

From: SeriousSchmendrick4428@aol.com
Subject: What the hell?
To: LoriSolomon6697@yahoo.com

So in a nutshell, Angela had one of her hyper-emotional, melodramatic outbursts last week about NOTHING. I told her to just chill out, and I haven't heard from her since. I just don't think that girl is happy unless there's some sort of quasi-tragedy going on in her life.

Anyway, you know what's interesting? Sometimes I'll wind up writing things that at the time seem completely relevant and perhaps even profound, but when I read them the next day they make no sense at all, either subjectively or even grammatically. However, there are times when I'll go back to it and suddenly it all makes sense for some reason. Does this mean I'm like two different people? Or that two different people are me? Or that I just can't stand two different people? Or that two different people are pulling me in opposite directions?

You should see the e-mail I recently sent to my friend Joe. It's like I'm just basically freaking NUTS, rambling and rambling about irrational nonsense almost like I'm doing a bad impression of William S. Burroughs. I wrote things to him like, "Take the bad laughs frozen loud without two quick outs for searing brain-sick lovelies, forcemeat gone gooey between the wind and the water with no time left to hold the poor peasants above the golden dome." Crap like that. What the hell was I TALKING about? I didn't take mushrooms or LSD or anything like that, and I didn't drink that much, either.

When I was younger I used to sleepwalk frequently, and I'm wondering if that's the kind of crap I'm doing again.

In a word, I'm worried. Last night, I swear to God I didn't do any major drugs except for drinking a few beers and smoking some weed. I remember going to bed perfectly well, too, but this morning when I woke up there was a DVD in my player that I have no recollection of watching, and there were e-mails that I sent to you and Joe- The both of you wrote things to me like "Are you on mushrooms" (that was yours, of course), and "Are you dropping acid again?" (that was his). His went on with a lot harsher accusations, though. He knows me better than you. It's messed up when you wake up to something like that and have no idea where it came from, especially considering that I DIDN'T take mushrooms OR acid.

Anyway, I don't know. Screw it. All I can say to you right now is to read whatever I write and take it with a grain of salt.

I might be sleepwalking and perhaps "sleep writing" again. I haven't had an episode of that crap in a while, though. I used to go to bed in one place and wake up in the next room, and sometimes I'd have pieces of paper with random attempts at surrealistic poetry strewn all over the floor around me. Sometimes I'd go to bed (relatively sober, mind you) and suddenly I'd wake up standing in my kitchen next to the microwave with a bag of Oodles-of-Noodles on the counter.

Well, we shall see. I shall monitor my situation. I shall smoke a joint now, drink a Sam Adams Winter Lager, and get my ass to bed.

Yours in madness,

Rutherford (a.k.a. Der Shcnitzen Haven)

Lori drove along the Mass turnpike, trying to admire the beautiful browns, pinks and yellows of the blur of sleepy trees guarding the roadside. Autumn was usually her favorite time of the year, and viewing the fall foliage at peak season was her main reason for taking the drive in the first place. Yet the scratching and clawing of anxiety-driven demons against the lining of her gut was making it impossible to appreciate it as fully as she would have liked to. She just couldn't understand why she seemed so unable to step out of her own way.

As the days swept past, their sunlight shone down on a growing inner strength while the moonlight of the evenings reflected a looming sense of tranquility. She threw herself into her studies with a passion and zeal that were invincible even in the face of all the continuing existing uncertainty. And she dreamt of endless possibilities, of finding real connections with real people, of brewing a fine mix of separateness and union and drinking up its intoxicating splendor. Life, at the moment, seemed full of promise. Life, at the moment, felt surprisingly *free*. She still thought of Nick, yet the uneventful passage of time was making his image more of an enigma to her than a painful obsession. And for that alone, life was perhaps the freest it had ever been.

Only one week into her newfound bliss, she received a phone message from Nick explaining to her that he had lost her e-mail address and asking that she start writing to him again. The sage inside her head shook with fear and cowered in the uncontrollable wrath of the toothless, drooling retread manning her heart. She sat down in front of the computer, hesitantly switched it on, and stared sadly at its slowly forming screen.

From: LoriSolomon6697@yahoo.com
mmmmmmm

yes?

From: NickWarren557@hotmail.com
mmmmmmm
when?????

She sighed loudly, the only evidence that her inner sage, although completely useless, was still conscious. She was so rarely placed in a situation where she knew she had complete control to make things better; where just a simple stroke of a few computer keys could make a colossal disturbance in her life disappear without a trace. Yet with all of her power something much bigger than her was keeping her from using it.

From: LoriSolomon6697@yahoo.com
eventually

From: NickWarren557@hotmail.com
why not tonight?

From: LoriSolomon6697@yahoo.com
busy

From: NickWarren557@hotmail.com
doin what?
where have my emails gone?
you usually write me a bunch
u mad at me?

From: NickWarren557@hotmail.com
so what sup

From: LoriSolomon6697@yahoo.com
no- not mad
just busy

From: NickWarren557@hotmail.com
why whats new?
what do you have planned for this evening?

From: LoriSolomon6697@yahoo.com
might exercise

From: NickWarren557@hotmail.com
exercise?
what we do or real exercise?

From: LoriSolomon6697@yahoo.com
REAL EXERCISE

From: NickWarren557@hotmail.com
ahhh well after give me a call on my cell phone

From: LoriSolomon6697@yahoo.com
o.k. to tell you i'm still busy

From: NickWarren557@hotmail.com
so what is the problem?
seems like your mad

From: LoriSolomon6697@yahoo.com
not mad
promise
just a lot on my plate right now

From: NickWarren557@hotmail.com
why whats wrong
pleeze tell
im here to help
ill put a big smile on those lips of yours

From: LoriSolomon6697@yahoo.com
you haven't gotten laid in a while, have you?

From: NickWarren557@hotmail.com
not since the last time i told you ... im honest!
so what about meeting and eating tonight

From: LoriSolomon6697@yahoo.com
i'm not in the mood

From: NickWarren557@hotmail.com
damn ... you're moody ...

From: NickWarren557@hotmail.com
so u gonna call me tonight to help you put a smile on
your face ... come on we can go to my house ... my
room ... my bed

The upsurge of attentiveness continued for several
days. The scales of dominance seemed to once again
be tipped in Lori's favor, yet she was not getting nearly
as perverse a pleasure out of the dance as she had
before. Perhaps her inner sage was not as
dysfunctional as she thought; perhaps it was trying to
protect her.

Yet when Nick sent her a photograph of himself,
sitting lazily in front of his work computer and looking
into the camera with a sardonic half-smile, she sensed
vulnerability in him that she never had before. Even if it
was just fleeting, as she was sure it was, he was
expressing a need for her. He was reaching out to her.
And he was getting dangerously close to wrapping his
fist around the goofy little retread that was licking his
wounds at the base of her heart.

From: LoriSolomon6697@yahoo.com
what am i supposed to do with this?

From: NickWarren557@hotmail.com
i dunno … just figured u might want it… u can look at me

Following a string of playfully seductive messages, Nick finally succeeded in breaking down her resolve- weak as it already was. On one chilly night at the radio station, she nestled in the soft, spacious back seat of his car and stared into the darkness ahead.

The shine from the car's dome light shadowed Nick's eyes to make them look like two black pits in a featureless face. He sat in the driver's seat with his hand impatiently clutching the steering wheel.

"It'll go off in a second," he said. His body was turned to face Lori, who sat rigid in the back seat.

After several minutes of uncomfortable silence, the air inside the car turned black. Lori kept her eyes fixed on a moonlit elm branch just outside the front windshield as Nick squeezed through the two front seats and positioned himself opposite her. He began removing his shoes, and gestured for Lori to do the same.

She knelt near him on the upholstery, her jeans rolled down past her calves and hugging her ankles. She continued to nervously stare out the windshield while Nick removed his boxer shorts and expectantly pushed his bare buttocks against the rear door. She lethargically lifted her blouse several inches above her panties, turned her head to face him, and continued raising the shirt up toward her chin.

"Take these off," Nick commanded, fingering the elastic of Lori's underwear and ignoring the bare skin that was revealed above her waist.

Lori took a deep breath and let her shirt fall back over her stomach. As she slid her panties past her knees, she felt the lukewarm air from Nick's car heater caress her thighs. She let Nick pull her hips toward his pelvis and push her down beneath him. Balls of sweat formed on his brow and dripped on Lori's cheek. He did not look at her. With his neck strained in an upright position, he alternated only between shutting his eyelids and glancing nervously out the back window of the car in search of intruders.

Lori turned her head to face the elm branch again. She continued staring at it until Nick finished and readily dressed himself. She did not take her eyes off of the branch until she was fully clothed as well, and even then she consciously kept it well within her peripheral vision.

As Nick turned the ignition key, silent and expressionless, fresh hot air blew against Lori from a car vent inches away from her chest. Still, there was a chill in the air that made Lori shiver, and a frigid wind that made the dry leaves on the elm branch sway.

"Do you miss having a girlfriend?" she asked, still staring into the tiny black forest ahead of his car.

"Sometimes yes. Sometimes no," he said. He pulled his jeans up over a hint of belly she didn't remember him having before.

"Could you ever see yourself as monogamous, Nick?" she asked.

"Yeah, I guess," he said. "If it all fell into place."

She was quiet. *If it all fell into place,* she thought. A familiar tingle crept up the sides of her neck. *And what would make it all fall into place, Nick?*

"I've been hurt by you before, and I'm afraid of getting hurt again," she said.

275

"O.K. Then just keep telling me no." He gave her a nervous smile, and started to tie one of his shoes. "Just keep saying no to me."

He brought her to silence again. She watched him make his loops and pull the strings taut on one shoe. He reached into the back seat to grab the other. It was obvious he was not going to deny the possibility of hurting her. Again.

"I can't do that," she said. "It doesn't work. It's an endless cycle with us."

He shrugged and smiled.

"What do *you* want?" she asked.

Still grinning foolishly, he opened his eyes wide and said, "*You* have to be the one to decide. Not me."

She said nothing for a moment. She started to gather her belongings and opened the car door. "You know, we have absolutely nothing in common."

He sat staring at her, with the same strange, contented look on his face. "We have sex in common."

She looked up toward the car's ceiling and blew a stream of air out of her mouth. "Even sitting here with you now is painful. Because I have no idea what to talk to you about." She turned her body and stepped outside the car. "We never have anything to say to each other."

He waited a few seconds before responding. "You have to just … not *think* so much about things. Just … go with the *flow*."

"I know," she said. "I think too much." She started to walk away. "Maybe I just try to make up for those around me." She lumbered across a patch of barely visible grass, and reached her own car only several feet away. She heard him start his engine and drive away, leaving her alone in the black emptiness of the night.

Chapter 25

Love is the triumph of imagination over intelligence
H.L. Mencken (1880-1956)

From: SeriousSchmendrick4428@aol.com
Subject: Re:
To: LoriSolomon6697@yahoo.com
I've been feeling pretty "bleh" lately, myself.
By the time you read this, I'm probably going to either have been fired or quit my job outright. On Friday afternoon, while I was sitting in the hospital with Jimmy for the THIRD straight week, I received a message from my agency that I had been "reported" by the hospital staff for sleeping on the job. I still can't believe this. It's not as if I'd brought a cot and a sleeping bag into the place. I was just sitting in a chair with my arms folded and I must have nodded off at the wrong point. Anyway, to make it short and sweet, this sort of infraction is historically used as a means to FIRE someone's unfortunate ass, and yet I don't give a crap. I've been instructed to report to the main office on Monday morning rather than go straight to the clinic like I usually do. What do you think the odds are that I'm going to set my alarm clock and make sure I make it to the office on time? DUH! NOT! On Monday, I'm not going to even attempt to get out of bed. Screw it. If I'm fired, then they can call me and fire me. I'm not disrupting my god damned day just to have my job handed to me with a handshake and a wink and a "seeya." I knew I was fired the minute I got that phone call on Friday. The whole thing SUCKS. Needless to say, I didn't bother staying at the hospital on Friday when I heard what was going on. I just got up from my chair and shook Jimmy's hand and said, "Well, man, I don't know if we're going to see each other any time soon. Take care of yourself." And I left.

I can't help but think this is all for the best. Without a kick in the ass to get myself in gear, I'd fall back into the day-to-day Jimmy thing and one or two or three years from now I'd be sitting here doing the same ol' god damned thing. Still, it bothers me. My parents both know what's going on and they're both ELATED that I'm quitting this stupid job once and for all. Or being fired... or whatever is happening.

It's one AM. I'm supposed to be at "work" in eight hours. I'm not even going to give them a chance to fire me. I'm walking into that building with a lengthy written resignation letter explaining why I can't work under such circumstances anymore. I'm not going to blame anyone or point any fingers or anything like that. I'm just going to be cordial and nice and say "good-bye" as best I can. What else can I do? Huh? What else?

"The sun is not yellow, it's chicken!"

Ponder that...

Rutherford

Lori sat across from Angela. She stared down at a full plate of fettuccini and picked at it with her fork.

"Eat, will you?" Angela said, smiling at her.

Lori started to chew on a chunk of garlic bread.

Angela wiped some grease off of the corner of her mouth. She pushed her plate of spaghetti a couple of inches toward the middle of the table. "I'm starting to get full," she mumbled, wiping crumbs off of her lap with a napkin.

Lori lifted her fork up and then placed it down next to her plate. She clasped her fingers together.

"Can I talk to you about Rutherford?" Angela asked.

"He said you both aren't talking... again."

"Rutherford's really messed up. He's really disturbed. Lori, I find him absolutely *evil*."

"He got caught sleeping during work. Did you know that? He might quit before they have the chance to fire him."

"I was actually thinking at one point about reporting him to the Department of Social Services, not necessarily on anything specific. Just to protest someone like him being in a position where he's taking care of someone else. He's shown that he isn't even capable of taking proper care of himself!"

"You know," Lori said. "Neither one of you seems to realize how your fighting affects me. Do you? And it's not just you. He pulls the same crap with me; making you seem like a lunatic and making me feel badly because of the pain you apparently cause *him*!"

"Well, what do you want me to do about it? Never mention his name to you? I don't think a case can be made that I was *ever* a lunatic in how I dealt with him. That's just his denial at work... and I think you know it. Are you and I both lunatics for seeing the truth?" She tipped her glass of ice water back into her mouth and stared hard at Lori.

Lori looked quietly back at her.

"Okay, bottom line. I just don't see how I've hurt Rutherford. All I ever did was *react* to the pain *he* caused *me*. End of story." She stabbed a pile of spaghetti and twisted it fast around her fork. She shoved more food than she was capable of eating quickly into her mouth, and tried chewing on it. She grabbed for a napkin and pressed it against her lips, and spit some of the spaghetti back out into it.

Lori was silent. She started to play with the dangling fringes of the tablecloth.

Angela pinched the edge of her plate. She pulled it closer to her, and then fingered a piece of garlic bread before slowly bringing it to her lips. "I *know* that Rutherford mistreated me *far more* than I ever

279

mistreated him. In fact, anything I ever did that caused him to label me 'pathological' or a 'lunatic' *was in reaction* to crap he pulled on me. I think he's finally seeing it the way it is, and that's why he's been apologizing up and down all over the place." She shut her eyes for a split second. "I guess what I'm confused about is, even though he's your friend, why wouldn't you have just taken a stand on *my* behalf when I first started to complain about him? Sometimes, even if someone is your friend, you have to be willing to tell them when they are being an ass. But, I'm getting the feeling that because you seem angry with *me* that you think I'm an ass too! And I haven't done anything but try to be a good, caring friend to Rutherford. I just feel like I can't win ..."

"Could you at least consider just distancing yourself from this guy who's upset you so much, so many times?"

Angela took a sip of water.

Lori continued, "Because it only ends up hurting me, to see you both hurting each other. That is, unless deep down you are enjoying the pain. And if that's the case, Angela, then I'm gonna have to ask you not to mention him to me again. Because the whole dynamic between you guys really disturbs me. You both tried friendship a few times, but realized that you're very different people who clash on a lot of different levels. It's not fun for me. Let's just leave it at that, okay?"

Angela put the glass of water to her lips again and tilted it slowly back. She swallowed hard. "I honestly don't think I'm looking to be abused, even 'deep down.' You forget. I got rid of this guy a long time ago, and I felt good about that. Then, after a conversation or two with you, I was convinced that *maybe* he'd changed enough for us to be friends. I tried, but quickly found out yeah, he'd changed, but not for the better. I think I've protected myself enough not to get nearly as hurt as before. But yeah, you're right when you say that he knows how to press my buttons and cause me pain. I don't know what to do now because I do have a heart, and he keeps pleading with me not to 'drop him' again!"

Lori rubbed her eyes with her fingertips and then moved her palms over her cheeks. For some reason her entire face had become itchy. "Look, I can't tell you what to do. I can only tell you that the way you two shoot the daggers at each other and then come running to me every time really hurts *me*. Can you see that? Can he see that?"

Angela set her glass down and slid it next to her plate. "Okay. I'm sorry for having done anything to hurt you with my relationship with him. I guess I just figured my complaints were totally justified, and couldn't see how that'd hurt you. I've never been able to make that connection, and I'm still finding it hard to understand."

"Look," Lori said. "I just feel like my friendship with Rutherford has been taking some pretty hard hits with all of this. I see it as being mainly his fault, for continuing this push-pull thing with you ... knowing he's pissing you off, and then apologizing, and then trying to suck you in again. But Angela, there's the 'batterer' and the 'battered.'" And after a while you have to take responsibility for being the one who keeps allowing herself to get sucked back in."

Angela smirked.

Lori smirked back. "I know what you're thinking. Just... give me a break here. You know I'm trying to work through my own problems."

They both ate silently. Lori paused in between tiny bites of her food. "I guess what I'm having a problem with is that there's a big difference between me listening to Rutherford go on with his false bravado crap and escapades with married women and harlots and

281

whoever, and me being put in a position where I have to hear how he's mistreating a good friend of mine. Do you want me to say something to him?"

"No, please don't say anything to him," Angela said. She pushed her chair out from underneath the table. "I feel that I'm only trying to do the 'right thing' with Rutherford. I've been trying to 'forgive and forget' when it comes to him, but right now I'm feeling that I should have just stuck with my original thoughts ... that he didn't deserve one single bit of my friendship. I don't know what to do, I really don't. I did offer to meet with him, face to face. He said there's a lot he wants to get off his chest."

Lori remained silent.

"This shouldn't be your battle," Angela said. "And I'm really sorry for having dragged you into this, and I'm feeling really, really bad."

Lori picked her fork up and started to spear a single strand of pasta that was dangling off the edge of her plate.

Angela glanced quickly up at her and then lowered her eyes to the table. Her tone softened. "Can we switch topics?"

"Sure," Lori said.

"Listen, I don't want to play mother and have you get all mad at me. But let me just say this. First of all, I think you are a *beautiful* girl. Not only that, I think you're unique-looking."

"Thanks," Lori said.

"But if you continue with your bad habits- The way you eat, no exercise ... you're going to start looking old before your time. As it is, and I say this with love, so don't get upset with me ... Every time I see you, you look drawn and tired. And you usually have dark circles under your eyes. Actually, you do right now."

Lori lifted her hand up to her face, and pressed her fingertips lightly against one of her lower lids.

"I always think to myself, 'God, if I had her looks, I'd do everything to preserve them.' As it is," Angela continued, "I don't think I am *bad*-looking... but I know I could look so much better if I were thinner and in better shape. I'm getting there, but damn it, I wish I'd started when I first started noticing the weight a few years ago. I just want you to take care of yourself. Trust me, time goes by faster the older you get, and you don't want to reach your mid-twenties and be staring at the reflection of a much older woman."

Lori kept her head bowed toward the dangling strand of fettuccini and continued to stab it mercilessly with her fork.

"I hope you're not upset with me," Angela said. "I'm only telling you this because I care about you."

"No, I'm fine," Lori said.

"Vitamins are the way to go, Lori," Angela said. "By just taking simple *vitamins*, my energy levels have *soared*. Even my mood's lifted up. I stopped taking Lexapro two weeks ago, and you know what? Don't miss it for a *second*. And I'm sure I'm doing my body a hell of a lot more justice. Who *knows* what those medicines end up doing to your brain after a while. Just take vitamins... as many as will fit in the palm of your hand, every morning. It'll transform you, Lori. I swear it will."

The waitress came by the table and began clearing away their dishes. Lori asked her to wrap up her virtually untouched platter of food, and watched the strand of pasta that she had mutilated fall off the edge of the plate into a heap on the tablecloth.

From: SeriousSchmendrick4428@aol.com
Subject: Hump the WHAT?

To: LoriSolomon6697@yahoo.com

Well, well, well. In a word, yesterday I tendered my resignation from my job. For two days I didn't call in or show up, and none of those clowns ever even called me to find out where the hell I was. In a word, I'm now jobless, penniless (except for a couple thousand dollars... which will disappear QUICKLY, I'm sure). And I've got this weird bruise on my left leg that I can't remember how it happened. Good grammar. If you can set me up with some broadcasting work that'd be great. Tell those guys at the station that you know a complete psycho who could revolutionize the radio world. Tell them I'm DANGEROUS. Tell them I'm wanted in several states for attempted murder, grand larceny, and dancing with a mailman. Speaking of "psychos," yesterday I got a call from Jill for the first time in I can't remember when. We were both busy at the time, but we're planning on having a long talk tonight. Actually, it was nice to hear her voice again. I wonder if this is destined to go anywhere. I'll always have a "soft-spot" for her, for whatever reason. I'd like to say "can we just skip the crap and hop into bed, for Christ's sake?" but I don't want to be too hasty or over-aggressive.

I will speak with thou soon.

Rutherford

Chapter 26

Even a small thorn causes festering
Irish Proverb

From: AngelontheAirwaves3254@hotmail.com
Subject: Re:
To: LoriSolomon6697@yahoo.com
Hey- I have lost TEN POUNDS in less than two weeks, just from being off Lexapro and on a new medication!!! I have a feeling the weight is going to fall off me, because a lot of it was "false weight." I also have tons of energy, like you wouldn't believe. Screw the vitamins! Give me meds instead any day of the week!!!!!!!!!!!!!!!!!!!!!!!!!!!!!!!!!!!!
Angela

From: LoriSolomon6697@yahoo.com
Subject: Re:
To: AngelontheAirwaves3254@hotmail.com
I'm on a swinging pendulum with you here. It wasn't that long ago that you were saying "screw the medications, just take vitamins." Why not wait a while and see what works for the long-term before you do a complete upheaval of your lifestyle? I've heard you talk about pounds just "melting away" a few times before, and losing five pounds here and five pounds there, only to have the weight come back again. I'm not sure I believe in any real magic formula when it comes to weight gain and loss, or that one thing is necessarily so much better than the other. I'd still take vitamins, exercise, and keep doing the things that you know are healthy for you.
Lori

From: AngelontheAirwaves3254@hotmail.com
Subject: Re:

To: LoriSolomon6697@yahoo.com

I was JUST KIDDING when I said "screw the vitamins; give me the medication!" The e-mail could not capture this... but I was actually MAKING FUN OF MYSELF!!!!! The fact that I am always looking for (and think I'm finding) quick fixes to all my problems is kinda humorous to me... So I was just poking fun at myself. Who knows if this will work? I think if I combine it with healthy eating habits and exercise, though, it has a good chance of working.

I thought you would "get" my joke, but apparently not. That's not your fault; like we've said a million times, e-mail is not the best way to communicate.

I do know that the Welbutran is making me feel better mentally than the Lexapro. I have some leftover Lexapro if you want it.

Love you!!!

Angela

From: LoriSolomon6697@yahoo.com
Subject: Re:
To: AngelontheAirwaves3254@hotmail.com

I'm so used to your intense, hair-raising, feverish focus on new pursuits, how in the heck am I supposed to realize you're kidding, you loon?

Well, I guess I'm off to bed. Did some reading for geography, will do the rest tomorrow morning. My studying schedule this week should be pretty manageable, so long as I give myself some breaks in between.

Talk to you sometime soon. Let me know when you'd like to try for another get-together.

Lori

From: AngelontheAirwaves3254@hotmail.com
Subject: Re:

To: LoriSolomon6697@yahoo.com
Please cut me some slack, will you? The ONLY reason I ever indulged in so-called "hair-raising, feverish focus on new pursuits" was because, after having been morbidly DEPRESSED for the past THREE YEARS, I was just completely desperate for something to ease the pain of my very existence. I was open to ANYTHING- be it drugs, vitamins, exercise, what have you. I will not hide the fact that I am STILL depressed, still searching, searching for something that will help me deal with the every day pain of survival.
Angela

Lori didn't understand what it was that drew some people to malevolence over and over again. She wondered if it could be the undeniable challenge of conquering something virtually unconquerable, and the thrill of the occasional victory, even if it was only temporary. Could those transient moments of glory be so powerful as to wash away all the plaguing memories of failure, generating a natural high like one gets from the rush of endogenous endorphins? If so, then she supposed it was no great secret as to why the moths continued to get burned by the same damning flame. Why the alcoholic kept stocking the liquor. Why the battered wife insisted on bailing her husband out of jail. Why she ...

From: LoriSolomon6697@yahoo.com
did you find the caricature i drew of you, under your calendar?

From: NickWarren557@hotmail.com
it's good. is it suppose to look like me?
well if it is u forgot my think piece!

From: LoriSolomon6697@yahoo.com
think piece?

From: NickWarren557@hotmail.com
i meant thick!

From: LoriSolomon6697@yahoo.com
i drew your head, didn't i?

It was the same inane dribbling that the two of them had turned into an art form. It was their characteristically weak attempt at witty banter that she felt was lost in the face of his seeming lack of depth, and her tendency to overanalyze. What, exactly, they both got out of their dizzying exchanges was a complete puzzlement to her.

From: NickWarren557@hotmail.com
just think of where my tongue is going to be

From: LoriSolomon6697@yahoo.com
i'm assuming inside your head

From: NickWarren557@hotmail.com
in my head plus …

From: LoriSolomon6697@yahoo.com
you haven't been laid in like … weeks now, right?
should i be taking out some form of insurance?

From: NickWarren557@hotmail.com
NO JUST MORNAL FUN SEX

From: LoriSolomon6697@yahoo.com
i just looked up the word "mornal" to see what it means
i couldn't find it

i'm taking out insurance

From: NickWarren557@hotmail.com
well it was misspelled … "normal"
don't be wise

From: LoriSolomon6697@yahoo.com
don't be dyslexic
i need a translator with your e-mails
SLOW DOWN!!!!!!!!!!!!!!!!!!!!!

From: LoriSolomon6697@yahoo.com
you might be gone for the day
but … did you call here?

From: NickWarren557@hotmail.com
YEAH I CALLED THERE
WHATS ABOUT TONIGHT?

He insisted on seeing her that evening, despite the fact that she had been stricken with a dry cough that was keeping her awake until the early hours of each morning. He was standing in the cold outside the radio station waiting for her, his hands digging into his pockets for warmth, a backpack over his shoulder weighing him down. She could see him walk slowly and cautiously over to the passenger side when she pulled her car near the curb.

"Didn't think you were comin,'" he said. He moved some of her textbooks out of his way and set them down by his feet.

"There's a lot of traffic," she said. Her voice was scratchy and broken.

"You sound really healthy." He smiled. "Not."

"I told you I was sick."

"What are we listening to?" he asked, pointing his chin toward the car's cassette player. A slow and smooth, smoky rendition of Kiss's "Rock and Roll all Night" was seeping through the car's stereo speakers.

"It's part of a mix that my friend Rutherford made for me," she said. She was relieved that he finally could hear music being played in her car that wasn't a complete embarrassment.

"This is just a nice, friendly visit," he said. He sat still in his seat and smiled at the open road ahead of them. "Just a friendly visit."

They drove for a little while without saying anything to one another. Maybe they really did have nothing in common, and it was possible that making conversation would never be as easy as peeling their clothes off. From what he described to her in terms of his actual experiences as well as fantasies, he seemed to know nothing of passion. He didn't seem to *want* to know anything of passion. He only dreamt about and engaged in the mechanics of sex, or perhaps he liked to think of it as the *adventure* of sex. She realized that she would probably never be anything other than the prop he so often treated her like, because that was all he seemed capable of seeing her as.

"So …" she began. "Do you ever see yourself settling down? Not too long ago you told me you could see yourself as monogamous."

He shrugged. "Nah. I dunno. I guess I like variety too much."

"What did Mona look like?" she asked. "I thought I saw her one night in Belchertown."

"Short reddish, blackish hair. Nice butt. C cup chest."

"Red highlights?" she asked. "What about her face?"

"Her face? Hmmmm … Tan. Nice smile," he said.

"How would you describe me?" she asked.

He winked.

"Come on," she said. "Give me a description like you gave for Mona."

"O.K.," he said. "Nice long hair, nice eyes, lips. I say B or C cup."

Nice eyes, she thought. *Nice long hair, nice lips*. For that quick, passing moment, Nick seemed to be suggesting that he saw her as slightly more than simply a warm orifice. She was a warm orifice with nice eyes, nice long hair, and nice lips. She supposed that as long as she was made to feel like an *attractive*, warm orifice, then she was a warm orifice with a healthy, nurtured self-esteem as well.

She drove Nick to his parked car at the Commuter Rail station. She watched as he began walking across the vast parking lot toward his car. She waited until he was little more than a sliver of motion in the far, dark distance, and then she started driving back toward the thruway alone.

From: LoriSolomon6697@yahoo.com
hope you like the key chains!
i left gifts for a few other people at the station, too

From: NickWarren557@hotmail.com
yeah they were cool thanks
i have a present for you

From: LoriSolomon6697@yahoo.com
what's that?

From: NickWarren557@hotmail.com
you'll have to unwrap it and find out

From: LoriSolomon6697@yahoo.com

ahhhh

From: NickWarren557@hotmail.com
when u want your present

From: LoriSolomon6697@yahoo.com
are you going to the xmas party tomorrow night?

From: NickWarren557@hotmail.com
yes hunny

    Lori was still clinging, restlessly grasping onto the shabby vestiges of what she knew deep down inside was slipping away. It seemed now to be mostly out of habit to wake up and send a few stimulus words off in haste through the computer, much as one gulps a hot cup of coffee or smokes a cigarette while scanning the morning paper. But there was still a twisted, lingering desire driving her to keep the connection alive, no matter how she tried to deny it or downplay her feelings. There was still the vision of lips pressed against lips, and flesh sliding against flesh, even if she knew the reality never even came close anymore to matching the fantasy.
    He loved to tease her about Angela, whom he still had not met in person. Lori couldn't bring herself to admit to him that Angela would rather spend her time squeezing pimples on the dysenteric ass of a wild gazelle than participate in an orgy with him in all his naked glory.

From: NickWarren557@hotmail.com
hehe
maybe ill have a fling with her ... lol

From: LoriSolomon6697@yahoo.com

that's fine with me
and you can go screw yourself, too

From: NickWarren557@hotmail.com
hehe settle down girl

From: LoriSolomon6697@yahoo.com
are you bored with only me as a partner?

From: NickWarren557@hotmail.com
not bored with you

From: NickWarren557@hotmail.com
so you wanna come over tonight after the party for
some good dirty fun

From: LoriSolomon6697@yahoo.com
so long as you don't gravely upset me

From: NickWarren557@hotmail.com
ahhh ok

Lori and Angela arrived at the party an hour and a
half after it had already started. Nick was standing with
his back to the entrance of the crowded restaurant. He
was wearing a gray knit sweater with rolled up sleeves,
clutching a bottle of beer.   Lori lightly placed her hand
on his hairy forearm and squeezed it.

"Well, hello," he said, raising his eyebrows and
turning to face her.

"Hi," Lori said. "Should you be drinking that?" she
asked him, pointing to the cream ale in his hand.

"One or two once in a while won't hurt me."

Lori nodded. "Angela? Get over here. I want you to
meet Nick."

"Who?" Angela was concentrating on buttoning her fire-red blazer with her cold, chapped hands as she approached him. "I'm sorry?"

"Nick," Lori repeated.

He chuckled.

"Oh!" Angela said. She reached for his hand and shook it. "You look different from how I pictured you."

"Is Helga or Burt here?" Lori asked him.

"Yeah, Burt's right over there," he said, pointing toward a group of people standing near a buffet table.

Lori walked over to Burt and gave him a big hug.

"Lori!" he yelled, throwing his arms around her. "How are ya?" He tossed his head back to move some long brown strands of hair out of his eyes.

"Fine, fine. Where's Helga?" she asked.

"Aah, she couldn't make it," he said. "Look at you... all dressed up!"

"Here," Lori said. She lifted some small gifts out of the pockets of her cloak. "These are for you guys."

"Thanks!" he said. He leaned toward her and whispered, "There's so much that I want to talk to you about. I was going to call ya, you know. The other day."

"Is everything all right?" Lori asked. She noticed that Angela and Nick were talking to each other a few feet away.

"Oh, yeah. No. Everything's fine." He drew hard on the end of his cigarette. "It's just that they're working us at the station to the bone now. And Helga, you know. Things with her, and the station, can get pretty intense sometimes, ya know?"

Lori nodded. She coughed into her gloves, which were still wrapped around her hands. The virus she had caught a week and a half earlier was still strangling her vocal cords and making her throat dry and her voice hoarse.

She slowly pulled her coat off, and then stood facing Nick. Her slinky, short-sleeved black dress suddenly felt foreign and odd against her skin. She peered up at him quickly, catching his gaze for only a second before nervously turning her head away.

She reached for one of many idle glasses of red wine on a nearby table. Burt tugged gently on her arm, and then guided her up a short flight of stairs to a quaint little alcove with sky blue-painted walls. They sat at a small, oval table with chairs overlooking a fire escape that led to some alleyway dumpsters.

Lori looked over her shoulder and realized that she couldn't see Nick anymore in the swarms of people below the stairs. Burt smashed his cigarette butt against a plate smeared with spaghetti sauce, and then pulled a fresh Winston out of a pack. While lighting it, he sucked hard on its end and blew a smoke ring into the air that wafted past Lori's nose.

"You know," she said. "I remember when we used to do bits together. There was one time I had such a splitting headache. Then you and I ended up laughing so hard that the headache just disappeared."

Burt smiled. "We had some good times," he said. "Came up with some good stuff."

Angela approached with a plate filled with noodles. She sat down and began picking at the pasta on her dish. "Did you get anything to eat?" she asked Lori.

"Not yet," she said.

"Eat! Will you? Jesus. That Nick is such a jerk. I didn't think I'd be able to get rid of him. He was just hanging around me ... and hanging around." Angela filled her mouth with a batch of noodles that were stuck together.

Burt continued to talk. Lori pretended to listen to him while looking out the window at a trash bin across the alleyway outside the restaurant. She pretended not to be irked by the thought of Nick preying on Angela as she stared at a piece of paper dangling from the edge of the dumpster and waving in the wind.

She returned to scouring the masses of people below their table, straining to see Nick. She politely excused herself, stood up and migrated to the buffet table, where she loaded up a plate with lukewarm Italian food. She searched the entire room, yet still did not see a trace of his gray knit sweater or the hairy arms that had jutted out from it.

He was gone.

From: LoriSolomon6697@yahoo.com
so...
you shamelessly flirted with Angela
and then disappeared
what is wrong with you?

Lori sent the e-mail off from her home computer. The wine that she drank at the party was doing nothing to tame the wild boar that once again was unleashed to wreak havoc in her brain. She silently crept into her bed and pulled her soft, patchwork comforter up around her shoulders. She thought back to the blur of beautiful autumn trees that she had been too impaired to enjoy as she drove along the lonely turnpike that one day. She wrapped the blanket tighter around her torso and nestled her head deep into her pillow, and she tried to distance herself just enough to realize how ridiculous all this really was.

From: NickWarren557@hotmail.com
ohh hehe oh well
that's me

From: LoriSolomon6697@yahoo.com

do you want it to be over?

From: NickWarren557@hotmail.com
im just kidding settle down

From: LoriSolomon6697@yahoo.com
i'm not kidding
apparently you want it to be over
otherwise you wouldn't have treated me the way you
did
guess what?
i finally want it to be over too

From: NickWarren557@hotmail.com
what ever i didn't treat you any way bad

From: LoriSolomon6697@yahoo.com
i thought we had made plans to see one another

She moved her chair backwards away from the computer with such force that it crashed into her bed frame. She had never before been so verbose with him in an e-mail exchange, never before expressed herself so fully to him. Up until then she had been sporting kid gloves, and had been reluctant to put up too much of a fight for fear of losing. Her long-standing angst had been due to her long-standing acceptance of which of them actually had the power. She had warily acknowledged which of them was the one to supply and sell the drug, and which of them was really the desperate addict willing to give up anything- even dignity- for even just a small sample of it.

From: NickWarren557@hotmail.com
oh ok whatever … lol

From: LoriSolomon6697@yahoo.com
why did you do that?
i just want to know

From: NickWarren557@hotmail.com
i didn't do anything

Angela had played a string of angst-ridden songs for her one night at Lori's apartment. Each successive song she played was angrier than the one before it, all obviously written by the most furious of women scorned.

"Listen to this," Angela had said to her, staring dreamily up at the ceiling while lying lethargically at the edge of Lori's bed. "Just listen …" She started singing along with the melody resounding from the speakers of Lori's stereo system. Her voice was clear and beautiful, and her eyes reflected the frustration of not being able to penetrate the impenetrable.

"Just listen," Angela repeated, losing herself in the music.

From: LoriSolomon6697@yahoo.com
Subject: Re:
To: AngelontheAirwaves3254@hotmail.com
For whatever reason, I am up at five AM.
While washing dishes after I got home last night from the party, Paul came to mind. And I thought, "I don't get it." And waking up this morning, I have to say that I still … just don't get it. I don't get why this has been so difficult for me. There'd been no guy on the planet with whom I'd gotten along so well, with whom I could talk so easily, with whom LIFE was just so EASY. Why, then, have I for so long been mesmerized with this other putrid schmuck?

I'm sorry I wanted to leave the party earlier than you, but in all honesty, I was feeling terrible ... about the mind games ... the fliration with you. Then he just left without so much as even saying good-bye.
Lori

From: AngelontheAirwaves3254@hotmail.com
Subject: Re:
To: LoriSolomon6697@yahoo.com
Hey Baby Cakes,
Nick REALLY wasn't flirting with me. It was just awkward between us because after all this time we finally met…and it was tough for me to know how to talk to him, or what to say. I was just trying to have a "normal" conversation with him… and getting off the subject of all the so-called women in his life. It was honestly just a boring as hell conversation. He made NO moves on me whatsoever. The only thing he said was that he wanted my phone number before the night was over … so that he could "harass" me with calls. But he never got it, so how much did he really want it? Lori, the guy is a player. But he's too much of a dink to be taken seriously. So that makes him a wannabe player. He's absolutely pathetic, and I just cannot figure out what redeeming qualities you see in him. First of all, you NEED to stop this e-mail crap with him. I know I'm just like you… and I HAVE indeed done what you are doing… but not for as LONG, I must say. I mean, the thing with Ted (the sleazy cameraman) lasted only a few months… the thing with Doug Wolfe (the older man who couldn't keep it up) lasted only a few weeks… and the thing with Rutherford, only two months. And while he still has an effect on me, there's none of this creepy erotic e-mail crap! This is zapping your precious energy, Lori. And I know that nothing I say in this e-mail is

going to make a difference. But I have to keep speaking my mind.

Anyhow, I have my own stressors these days. I keep thinking my new job at Springfield's Channel 6 is going to be taken from me once the network realizes they don't want an ugly, fat girl on their airwaves. I'm having a bad self-esteem day, Lori.

Your L.L./S.F.,

Angela

It was the next day. Sitting on Lori's computer were a series of delayed e-mail interactions that had obviously occurred the previous morning. She had gone to sleep the night before assuming that Nick was not going to even attempt conjuring up a pacifying explanation for her, consumed either with sheer denial or the intoxicating power that comes with sadistic manipulation.

From: NickWarren557@hotmail.com
no i was just tired and i had to catch a train that's why i left quick … sorry

There was only a trace of blood lining the infrastructure of the stone that was Nick Warren. Although it was not nearly enough to sustain life, Lori was still touched to know that it was there at all.

From: LoriSolomon6697@yahoo.com
i overreacted, and i'm sorry

From: NickWarren557@hotmail.com
yeah you better be …

From: LoriSolomon6697@yahoo.com
you still left without saying good-bye

From: NickWarren557@hotmail.com
oh im sorry … it will never happen again
you feelin better

From: LoriSolomon6697@yahoo.com
still have a little bit of a cough … and a raspy voice

From: NickWarren557@hotmail.com
hehe. how do you feel about some ... to go in your ...

From: LoriSolomon6697@yahoo.com
i honestly don't know how i feel

Days elapsed with only scarce communication between the two of them. The few exchanges they had were only mildly seasoned on either end with subtle innuendos of desire. There were the typical upsurges of overt passion-driven intensity on Nick's end, followed by cautious yet convivial replies on Lori's end. And these upsurges, and the sweet anticipation they stirred, were followed by days and nights of disheartening empty silence and echoing distance.

Chapter 27

When there is no enemy within, the enemies outside
cannot hurt you
African Proverb

From: SeriousSchmendrick4428@aol.com
Subject: Atomic dump
To: LoriSolomon6697@yahoo.com

So I spent most of last night scrounging around for scraps of wood to burn in my stove for some HEAT in this dump, in addition to taking frequent naps where I'd usually wake up screaming in horror when faced with the realization of how my life is in complete chaos right now. Check this out:

Dear Rutherford,

It has been reported to me by your supervisor Ashly Wood that you have failed to report to work. We were also informed that while you were working with an individual (they're referring to Jimmy here), you were reported sleeping on the shift.

Your position with the agency has been terminated for violating TTS's Personnel Policies and Work Rules.

TTS's Personnel Policies Section #301; Immediate Discharge;

#8 Repeated absenteeism;

#14 Acting in a way which damages the reputation, prestige, or credibility of the Organization

#22 Other conduct which in the sole discretion of TSS, continued employment would be contrary to the Organization's best interest.

TSS's Work Rules:

#40 Sleeping on duty is prohibited, unless permitted for "asleep overnight" employees. Employees shall be awake, alert, and attentive at all times when on duty.

Rah Rah Rah... That's basically it. I received this in the mail the day after I handed in my resignation notice. Two years of working for those dickheads and they send me a letter like this in the freaking mail?

Oh, well... I really don't care. "Repeated absenteeism?" In the two years that I worked for those bastards, I think I called in sick like TWICE. Is that "repeated absenteeism" in your opinion? "Other conduct which in the sole discretion of TSS, continued employment would be contrary to the Organization's best interest?" I wonder if they're talking about my rampant, obvious, and continued drug use. They knew I was doing coke and drinking whiskey on the job as far back as a year ago, but NOW it's a problem! I'm speechless, precious.

I must go to bed now. I can't believe what I've just read...

Rutherfugged

Angela and Lori sat across from each other in a darkened booth in a Chinese restaurant. Despite the poor lighting, Lori could see that the walls had been painted an emerald green color that matched the upholstery they were sitting on. Candles lit in dangling copper holders and raging fires from the centers of widely distributed Pu Pu platters cast enough light for Angela and Lori to be able to see their menus. And just enough light was also shining down on a furrow in Angela's brow for Lori to sense that there was some kind of trouble brewing.

"I want to apologize for dragging you into all of my ups and downs with Rutherford," Angela said. She gently placed her reading glasses down on the table and lowered her menu. "I think I've made the mistake of dwelling too much on his negatives and not enough on his positives."

"Why? What's going on?"

"We were together all day yesterday, talking. He was like an angel. I wasn't feeling well, and he knew it, and he rubbed my back, and my feet... He was like a nursemaid. I think he's a really good-hearted, caring soul. And the mistake I've been making is painting all these unfair pictures, based on things I should have been able to take in stride and not go to pieces over."

Lori nodded, and took a sip of ice water.

"Now. That having been said," Angela continued. "Do I think he's immature and irresponsible and lazy at times? Absolutely! But every day I see him trying harder and harder to grow up and be responsible. And I *always* praise him when I see signs of maturity. People respond so much better to praise when they do the right thing, than criticism when they do the wrong thing, you know? I mean, he's so smart and talented, yet he isn't doing *anything* with it. I think he gets so overcome with everything that he *should* be doing to get himself back on track, that sometimes he just doesn't do anything constructive- just rots in his apartment, or sometimes at the lake, just pissing time away. All I can do is be there for him as a friend."

Lori nodded again, and took another sip of her water.

"We've been getting along so great, Lori. I mean really great. We spent the most incredible day yesterday. I'm telling you that when it was over we both felt like crying. But ... I just feel like such a fat *cow* when I'm with him. And it's like, it has *nothing* to do with the way he treats me. Nothing whatsoever. He tries to make me feel like the most beautiful, sexiest girl in the world. And there's no way he could be faking it because of the way he constantly looks at me and touches me. So... *What is wrong with me*? Why can't I just accept this guy's love and not question it? *That's* really the issue here, Lori. I've got some big problems. Sometimes I think I have issues that I'm not even aware of."

Lori shrugged, and took another sip of water. "Don't know what to tell you, Angela," she said.

Angela stared at her.

Lori shrugged again. "I mean I just don't know what you want me to say about this."

"Why don't you just tell me what you think?" Angela said, the furrow in her brow deepening.

"I'm in no position to make any judgments here. Just pay close attention to your instincts, I guess. And go from there."

The waitress appeared and took their orders, and then their menus. Angela shot an angry look at Lori.

Lori looked back at her, perplexed.

"Lori, I just want you to know that it hasn't gone unnoticed that you haven't exactly been your 'warm, friendly' self toward me lately."

"What do you mean?"

"You seem pissed off at me a lot of the time. And I don't think it's my imagination, because you never used to be this way. Maybe I just shouldn't talk to you anymore about Rutherford? I mean, I have enough tension in my life without adding more to it."

"Angela, you know, earlier today at home, I played back some old voice-mail messages that you left. There was one where you sounded really upset, and were saying how you didn't want to keep in touch with Rutherford because the fights between both of you were too painful. If Rutherford *didn't* bother you the way he has a tendency to, then I wouldn't have anything to say. Plus, his life is so up in the air right now."

"But I really think he's changing, Lori. I mean, I know he's going through a lot, but I think it's all for the better. The way it looks at this point is that we're definitely *together* and happy. I mean, I'm keeping my guard up, and I still get insecure. But that's all in my head, and has nothing to do with the way he treats me."

"What about the drugs, Angela? What about his drug use?"

"He and I have talked about that. He's gonna get help. He wants help, and I want to help him get that help. Look, Lori, I *know* what it's like to have an addictive personality. I know what it's like to feel broken inside and to reach out for things that make you feel intact, even though it's those same things that tend to damage you even further."

The waitress arrived with cokes in her hands. Lori pushed her glass of water to the side and clutched the glass of soda that was placed in front of her. She covered the tip of the straw with her lips and began sucking fiercely on it.

"We went back to his place, Lori, where he lit scented candles, and we made love for literally hours. It was just beautiful."

Lori looked up from her coke. She stared hard into Angela's eyes.

"What's wrong?" Angela asked.

"Nothing," Lori mumbled, lowering her eyes toward her straw and placing her lips over its tip again.

"I just feel *so good* when I am with him, Lori. This may sound like a small thing, but I love that he actually laughs at my jokes! When I was with Hugh, a few years back, it was like no one could be funny except *him*, and there were times when I could see him literally trying *not* to laugh if I said something funny. He had to be superior over me in every way. Rutherford seems so supportive of me... in every way. I just hope it lasts. I am in heaven when I am with him, Lori, and I hope so much that things continue to go well."

"Food's here," Lori said, moving her drink to one side. A plate of orange chicken was set in front of her, with a side bowl of fried rice. She started to eat.

"Lori, I have never in my life had such an intense spiritual and emotional connection with *anyone*. Not even close. And it's the 'emotional' closeness that I am certain makes the sex so off the scale. We're spending the weekend together. His roommate is going away for the weekend, so I'll be staying over there Saturday night."

Lori continued to eat.

Angela sighed. "You know, I can't help but take your silence a little personally. I think that *you* think I'm headed for a big *fall*. And no matter what I say to you about him, and all the change I see happening, all the change that I know is well in motion, that's what you think, isn't it?"

"You want everyone to ebb and flow with your moods and situations," Lori said. She pitched her fork in the center of a piece of chicken and let it fall to one side. "And to forget the negative things you've said when you're feeling positive, and to disagree with the positive things you've said when you're feeling negative."

"I don't want everyone to *ebb and flow* with my moods and situations. I reject that statement completely," Angela said.

"You want honesty. I give you honesty. And you don't want to hear it. Tell you what. I won't say anything to you unless I know it's what you want to hear. But then you can't blame me for not being a true, honest friend to you when I think you're headed for trouble, or might want to hear a different perspective on a situation. You can't have it both ways, and I'm getting a little tired running from one end of the spectrum with you to the other, not knowing which end you want/need me to be on!"

Angela sat, quietly staring down at her food. She rocked an egg roll back and forth on her plate with her fork.

"Do you understand where I'm coming from?"

Angela continued to play with the egg roll.

"Look. Relationships are tricky," Lori said. "And what one might think will work might not, and what one might think won't work, will. What do I know about it? The last thing you need is the input of a complete idiot like me."

"I'm trying to tell you, Lori, that Rutherford and I *are* together, and are very happy," Angela said. "But I *do* still struggle with general relationship issues and not feeling *good enough*. It's *never* been easy for me in a relationship... All of my relationships with guys have been nothing short of disasters. Part of that's because the guys I've been attracted to have been insecure and abusive. But the other part of it's *me* and my insecurities and issues that make it so tough for me to just *settle down*."

"I think if a person can let their guard down, just enough, it's possible to feel love for just about anyone," Lori said. "Even people who have hurt you."

"That sounds like pretty *evolved* thinking on your part."

"I just think that if more people saw life for what it really is ... and realized that it's not forever, it'd be easier to forgive and forget. It'd be seeing the big picture. We're all just these sorts of pathetic creatures thrown into this bizarre realm, filled with all kinds of weird forces and wacky creations, for reasons that are completely beyond our ability to know, or probably to even understand."

Angela reached over the table, tilted Lori's glass of soda, and peered inside. "You just ordered a coke, right?"

"I think you'd be a lot happier if you looked at life a little differently."

"I can't ... actually, I *won't* forgive and forget when it comes to anyone I know who's hurt me intentionally. And why should I? Why would I?"

"Because there's just so much more to it, I think, than you're allowing yourself to see," Lori said.

"Well what about that Ulf Fucher guy you used to complain to me about? You're telling me that your friend Pista would be willing to *forgive* and *forget* when it comes to someone like him, with everything you told me that went down between the two of them? I remember you telling me that Ulf guy was nasty even to you! And you were just a summer intern! No threat to him at all!"

"I had actually left a present for him, on his desk, before I left the lab."

"Lori..." Angela shook her head in disbelief. "He didn't deserve a *gift* from you! He didn't deserve *anything* from you!"

Lori shrugged.

"What did he do, after he saw he got a gift from you?"

"Nothing. I mean, he didn't *return* it, or anything like that. I didn't find it in the trash. So I'm assuming he accepted it."

"But he didn't thank you for it," Angela said.

"No, but giving him the gift made me feel better, knowing that I at the very least tried to get him to see that there are people who mean well out there."

Angela shook her head.

"I'm sure he's got his reasons for being a prick," Lori said. "I'm not saying they're necessarily *good* reasons, but they're his. Everybody's got their own story to tell that makes them who they are." Lori's throat was getting dry. She took a sip of her soda.

"I'm sorry, but … None of what you're saying makes any sense to me whatsoever." A tiny bead of sweat glistened on Angela's temple.

"I just like the idea of trying to make a bad situation ... not so *bad*. What's wrong with that? I can't change who he is or what he's done to people he's worked with. But I can let him know, in my own way, that things don't have to continue being the way they are."

"I think it's all well and good to want to 'rise above' peoples' bad behaviors. But it's another thing to actually give them gifts when they've mistreated you. Jesus was all about 'turning the other cheek,' but he didn't give people presents after they'd 'sinned.' He just told them he'd forgiven them and that they should try not to sin anymore. I'm not getting all religious on you here. I'm talking about how we ... collective 'we,' including you and me who tend to be too nice to people who've hurt us ... should deal with nasty people. Mainly to honor ourselves, but also to show those who've offended us that we respect ourselves too much to be taken advantage of. In other words, by rewarding these people, we're actually 'dissing' ourselves. And doggonit, *we* are just as valuable as *they* are! Know what I'm getting at here?"

Lori shrugged.

Angela took her napkin and patted the side of her head with it. She lifted her glass of soda, brought her straw to her mouth, and finished her drink in one sip. "Ulf didn't *like* you, Lori. I just don't understand your motive here unless you have this need to be accepted by everyone you come in contact with. You told me you gave Nick a gift for Christmas, and I think it was an equally dishonest, selfish... and even *manipulative* thing to do. It's like you're trying to buy their love. Why do you feel you need these people in your life?"

"I don't regret anything I've done, Angela," Lori said. "And I don't feel like debating about it. This conversation's over." Lori stood up and swept the check off the table. She fished frantically in her purse for enough money to cover the bill, and tossed it carelessly next to a poorly lit desert menu propped up as the table's centerpiece.

Angela trailed Lori closely as she made her way past tables and booths and flew through the front entrance of the restaurant. Once outside in the parking lot, Lori began searching for her car.

"Lori, just because I don't understand where you're coming from on this doesn't mean it has to turn into a big fight," Angela said. She peered past Lori's shoulder in search of her own vehicle. "Can't we just agree to disagree, and leave it at that?"

"I'm not dishonest or manipulative ... or whatever it was you called me," Lori said, thrusting her car key into the front door lock. She wondered how anyone could be so blinded by their own misery as to rebuke even the most humble attempts to see the positive over the negative. Were Angela's wounds so deep that she had crossed over to the dark side, crusading against all and any who reminded her of how horribly flawed this world can be? If true, then Lori could understand how Angela would be drawn to someone like Rutherford, who was on his own eternal hell bent crusade, warranted as he believed it was from all the injustices bestowed on him over the years.

"Lori, I just can't help but be really against *rewarding* people for bad behavior! You and I... We've *both* just been through *so much*, and I think we give far more than we get, and I just can't..."

"Angela, I don't see where you and I have been through *so much*. Fighting a terminal disease is going through *so much*. Being on welfare while trying to support a family is going through *so much*. Getting your ass blown away overseas in a war is going through *so much*. I just don't see the purpose of going through life waving the white flag of surrender and playing the ultimate victim all the time."

"I don't think it's fair to minimize the rejection and cruelty that you and I have gone through," Angela said. She clutched her purse tightly and began walking away from Lori, toward her car.

"It hasn't been *that bad* for me, Angela!" Lori yelled. "I wish you'd stop grouping us together as having had the exact same horribly traumatic experiences in life!"

"Well I don't think that you and I... or you and I and *Rutherford* ...would get along as well as we did if we *didn't* share similar experiences in life," Angela said. "And while we're on the subject, I want to tell you how hurt I am that you've been anything but supportive of everything I've told you about him tonight."

"You two had *one good time* together, Angela, and a whole bunch of really *horrible* times. Can't you see that? You seem to be able to see with like *laser vision* all the doom and gloom hovering over just about everything that *I* do in this lifetime... I'm surprised that this one is escaping you. Rutherford just lost his job... Maybe he's feeling extra needy right now, or maybe he's just lonely. I think that you just might want to give this a little *thought* first before you draw any rock hard conclusions about where all this is going."

Angela looked at Lori as though she had just sprouted goat horns and a hog's snout with "666" branded into her forehead. She backed away from her slowly, and continued to inch her way toward her car. "I don't have the emotional backbone for this," Angela said, quickening her backward pace. "I can't confide things in you only to have you come back with thoughts or advice that are damaging."

"Damaging?" Lori said. "Now what I say to you is damaging, huh? Look, the way I see it, Angela, is that you don't just *invite* people into your problems. You *drag* them in, and then you push them into a corner as to what they can, can't, should, or shouldn't say to you depending on what kind of *mood* you're in. But that's after you criticize them for not *predicting* what kind of mood you're in before saying something to you that doesn't jive with what you *wanted* or *expected* them to say!"

"Oh, oh!" Angela said, with her face suddenly strangely contorted. "Okay!" she screamed hysterically, waving her hands at Lori. "Good night!" she yelled, almost with a melody, as she disappeared in the front seat of her car. She pulled the vehicle out of the parking lot with vigor, the exhaust shooting out violently from behind and dissipating in the air almost as quickly as her car disappeared out of sight.

Chapter 28

A clear conscience is a soft pillow
German Proverb

The days and nights began to unfold, long and void, filled with nothing more than the silence of abandonment. Within every hour that ticked away, there were at least one or two moments colored either by hopeful longing that Lori would hear from Angela, or the hollow despair of believing she had lost her forever. She knew that she was just as drawn to Angela, and just as drawn to Rutherford, as apparently they were to each other. She also knew that what she was drawn to in Angela and Rutherford was similar to what she was drawn to in Nick. She had her own opaque darkness, and her own deep wounds that just wouldn't seem to heal, and there was a peculiar, almost shameful, comfort in knowing that she wasn't the only one harboring them. All the same, she felt a peculiar, almost shameful, need to try to comfort those who she knew harbored these same deep wounds.

From: LoriSolomon6697@yahoo.com
Subject: Re:
To: AngelontheAirwaves3254@hotmail.com
Angela,
I never wanted to upset you to the extent that I did the last time we had talked. Toward the end of that conversation, you had said that you felt the advice that I had been giving you was "damaging," and that was at least part of what I had reacted to. Up until then, I thought I had been helping, not hurting, by trying to be there when you needed someone to talk to, and I had tried to keep an open mind with the things you confided in me, and tried to keep my opinions somewhere in the

neutral zone. I'm not sure, as time went on, and I saw how upset you would get, and how often you would seem upset, if my opinions ended up staying so neutral. I guess I got too emotionally involved in what you've been going through, and more than anything I didn't want to see anyone get hurt.

I've been feeling badly that I never got the chance to explain myself. I'm sorry if I made matters worse- but I really didn't mean to, and I need for you to know this.

Lori

From: AngelontheAirwaves3254@hotmail.com
Subject: Re:
To: LoriSolomon6697@yahoo.com

Lori,

I appreciate your comments. But really, all things considered, I just can't continue in this friendship any longer. It's not just a few isolated incidents; it's a lot of things. Seems as much as we both try NOT to hurt each other, we end up doing just that. I don't want to analyze things anymore; we both did the best we could. It's just time to admit that the relationship doesn't work, and just throw in the towel before things get worse.

I wish you only the best in life.

Angela

It was a heavy blow aimed right at Lori's lower gut. She stared at the computer screen for a few moments, hoping to see the words on the screen turn more amicable, and less absolute. Yet, if anything, the words became more direct, more callous, and less forgiving with each unfolding second.

The sharp-shooting pain that she was feeling in her stomach was similar to the pain she had felt many times over in the past with Nick. Yet this pain curiously seemed to be much stronger. It clawed even deeper inside of her; it scratched the lining of her intestine with pointier, longer nails, and left behind deeper, bloodier gashes. Lori had really gotten to *know* Angela, and Angela had really gotten to *know* Lori. They had shared an intimacy that had never been muddied by pulsing testosterone or dizzying pheromones. They had given to and taken from each other freely, unabashedly, clear-minded and strong-willed. They had formed a bond.

Lori realized then that her world could be turned just as tumultuous and nauseating by a female as by a male. Angela was showing the same eerie ability as Nick to swing from all to none, in one detached bat of an eyelid. It was a similar hypnotic wave of scorching hot intensity followed by frosty estrangement.

But there was one difference.

This was Angela.

This was not Nick.

From: AngelontheAirwaves3254@hotmail.com
Subject: Re:
To: LoriSolomon6697@yahoo.com
Dear Lori,
My mom told me you called, and are sending a doll. Thank you in advance, although I cannot have any dolls in my room with me because the cats would tear them to shreds. Don't quite understand why you are doing this, Lori ... I mean, not letting go of our friendship. It is not just I who has been hurt by you; you have also been hurt by me. And it finally became painfully clear to me that we just don't communicate properly. There's been way too much misunderstanding and hurt feelings as a result. Why would you want to continue this?
It feels like in some ways we bring out the worst in each other, and end up inadvertently causing each other a

good deal of unnecessary anguish. I have of course missed you over the last several weeks ... But a part of me has also felt RELIEF not having to worry about getting hurt by you, or being the one hurting you.

What do you propose doing about this? I am open to anything, but I also feel very guarded right now. Scared is more to the point. I do NOT, I repeat, DO NOT want to open myself up to getting hurt again.

Angela

From: LoriSolomon6697@yahoo.com
Subject: Re:
To: AngelontheAirwaves3254@hotmail.com

Dear Angela,

I hate whenever I upset you, and I know you feel the same about me. And I'm not sure if we can get past this or not. But what I do know is that I have come to care very deeply about you, and have considered you to be one of the closest friends I've ever had. A lot has to do with how much you've been willing to share with me, and lean on me as a friend.

The bottom line is all I've ever wanted to be is a good friend to you in return. The love is there; the caring is there. I've been so happy that we've gotten to know each other and that the friendship has developed. But for a while now, I really haven't known what it is that you need from me, and what I can do to be there for you without upsetting you at the same time.

Now I'M the one putting it all into words in a stupid e-mail, but I know if we met face to face I wouldn't be able to put the words together the way I am now. I still really would like to talk to you in person, and see if we can pick up the pieces here. And I'll leave you with this: Although I feel that I've gotten to know a lot of people over the years, it's a rare few that I feel I can really connect with. You, my dear, have been one of those

rare few, crazy as things seem to be and get between us at times. And that's why I'm having such a difficult time letting go. I see all the good, as well as the bad. I guess I've been wishing that you could see the same.
Lori

From: AngelontheAirwaves3254@hotmail.com
Subject: Re:
To: LoriSolomon6697@yahoo.com

I think what happened, Lori, is that you (and probably me, too, at times) just went too far with the "tough love" and crossed into mistreatment. During our last conversation, you had the complete audacity to accuse me of "dragging" my friends into my problems! That's when I knew I had to just walk away and refuse to listen to any more verbal attacks from you. Lori, let me take this opportunity to remind you that YOU HAD ASKED, LITERALLY BEGGED ME, TO CALL YOU AND TALK TO YOU ABOUT MY PROBLEMS, BEFORE TURNING TO SOMETHING SELF-DESTRUCTIVE LIKE DROWNING MY SORROWS IN ALCOHOL. I finally took the risk of calling you a few times when I was down and out (instead of drinking), not feeling in the least like I was "dragging" you into anything because you had made it so clear that you WANTED to be of help ... only to have my weaknesses thrown up at me with the accusation you made that day. I felt myself FILLED with regrets for having opened up to you and made myself so vulnerable to you. I also felt like you had NO RIGHT to lump all of my friends together, making it seem like everyone in my life felt "dragged" into my problems. None of my friends feel that way. Believe me, I asked them all after that. And they thought it was horrible that you would say such a thing to me.

I honestly felt that, as much as you claimed to want to make me happy, sometimes you would deliberately cut me down to size to make me feel awful, and even ashamed of myself.

So ... That's what I mean when I say that I really think you went well beyond "tough love" into a realm that only had the effect of plunging me into an even deeper depression than before a conversation with you.

Angela

From: LoriSolomon6697@yahoo.com
Subject: Re:
To: AngelontheAirwaves3254@hotmail.com

Dear Angela,

Thanks for opening up a dialogue with me. I wish that you could have explained to your friends that my comment (stupid as it was, and it WAS stupid) came after you referred to my advice as having been damaging. My reaction totally sucked, and I wanted to apologize for that as soon as the words flew out of my mouth. At some point in time, I'd like to just talk to you. Go to a restaurant. Eat, laugh, and just be friends. Maybe lay off the advice for a while. That doesn't mean that I don't want you to talk to me, and confide things in me. That's what's made our friendship so special- and GOOD. But maybe I'll be a better friend to you if I just listen to what you're saying, instead of feeling like I have to advise you on things, and maybe you'll be a better friend to yourself if you believe in yourself enough to trust your OWN advice. You're a much stronger, wiser person than you give yourself credit for being. And I'm just one of many fools on this big ol' ship!

Lori

From: AngelontheAirwaves3254@hotmail.com
Subject: Re:

To: LoriSolomon6697@yahoo.com

Lori, look. I really never wanted to end the friendship. I just wanted to end the pain that we were both (unwittingly) causing each other. I never thought we wouldn't EVER be friends again. It just seemed that the BOTH of us had overstepped each other's boundaries too many times, and I just found myself unable to cope with it any longer. Looking back, I know I over-reacted. But I was in a VERY fragile place at that point, and the last thing I needed (as I'm sure you can understand) was a close friend throwing accusations at me, and making me feel even guiltier than ever. I can understand how my comment about your saying things to "damage" me could have upset you greatly. I realize that by getting hysterical, I also denied myself the opportunity to explain what I'd meant by that. All I meant was that sometimes friends, even with the best of intentions, can say things to exacerbate a situation and cause even more depression and/or anxiety. I want to get a therapist to AVOID this sort of thing. Therapists are trained to know what to say and what NOT to say when a client is going through a hellish time. And even therapists can make mistakes and cause more harm than good! I never meant for you to think that EVERYTHING you'd ever said had "damaged" me. That is FAR from the truth. Much of your advice and counseling has been VERY helpful, and I appreciated it greatly! It just seemed to me that once you started to think you needed to give me the "tough love" approach, you got carried away with that and crossed some invisible line into what I felt was mistreatment. You were literally turning into a "Lori" I didn't know or understand anymore. And I just did not know how to react. I wanted the OLD Lori back!! I can take an occasional "kick in the ass," but it started to feel like you were putting your whole foot up there- and it was starting to hurt!

I feel the same way as you about knowing a lot of people, but feeling there are only very few that I can truly "connect" with- you being one of them. I just want us to figure out how to capitalize on that part of our relationship without getting into a lecturing mode ... or assuming things about each other that may not be accurate.

By the way, I only told two friends- Judy and Eileen- what happened between us. And their feelings were that you and I probably both said things we didn't mean in the heat of the moment, and that we would be friends again when the dust settled. They also both told me that you probably hadn't really meant that you'd felt "dragged" into my problems, and that I shouldn't feel that I had been some kind of burden to you. They also know that we're "talking" again, and they've been encouraging me to try to work it out ... because they know how much I care about you and how much the friendship has meant to the both of us over the last several years. So please don't think anyone hates you or thinks that you are a jerk. Quite honestly, Lori, I think we have BOTH acted like jerks to each other at certain points. And I just want that crap to stop, that is all. We both need to be a lot gentler with each other. We are both highly sensitive people, and that needs to be handled carefully, you know?

Angela

From: LoriSolomon6697@yahoo.com
Subject: Re:
To: AngelontheAirwaves3254@hotmail.com

I'm feeling a lot better. Honestly, I had been really down and out since our argument. I mean, really depressed. My reaction to everything made me very aware of the fact that I really don't rebound well at all from setbacks. This is another reason why our argument hit me so hard, as well as the possibility that the friendship was over. I want to be there for you when you're feeling this way- because I understand, and can really relate. Our friendship gives me this weird feeling of security, like there's someone else out there who "knows."

I really do feel sometimes like I'm in a "blind leading the blind" situation, because I wrestle with a lot of doubts and confusion about things all the time. I don't feel like I'm in a position to be doling out advice to anyone- ESPECIALLY when it comes to relationships! Relationships are just so unique to the people that are in them ... Also, I'm majoring in biology, not psychology. I might as well be Lucy Van Pelt with a booth taking nickels from little kids in the middle of a sidewalk.

Anyway, glad we're on the road to recovery.

Lori

Chapter 29

*All the art of living lies in a fine mingling of letting go
and holding on*
Henry Havelock Ellis (1859-1939)

Angela breathed heavily into the phone. "Lori, I don't know what to do about Rutherford. I've just been dealing with *so much* of his crap lately. I mean, things *were* good for the most part, but we'd have at least one good fight a week- either about money, or because he wouldn't arrive or call on time. Or because he'd call to tell me he'd be late at the same time he was *supposed* to show up. It's just been one thing after another with him. Lori, the last few times we were together, I was so disgusted with him that I had absolutely no sexual desire. I had to *force* myself to make love with him."

"I'm sorry you're going through a rough time," Lori said.

"Let me tell you what happened last week when I visited him in Portsmouth. He was supposed to meet me at seven-thirty. So he called me at seven-forty-five to tell me he was just leaving his parents' house, which was an hour away from the museum we were going to. He had every stupid, inane excuse in the book for not calling me earlier... Like sitting with his parents' kitchen clock to his back. Or leaving his cell phone in his car. And on and on it goes. Then he tried to turn the thing around to blame *me* for not being more understanding! This, after I'd gone out of my way to get tickets for us. We got into a screaming match at the museum ... I told him I just wanted to slap some sense into him, and he said he'd just slap me right back. I swear it was ugly and evil. I'm seriously thinking that this might be a good time to just 'cut my losses' and get out. I've been so consumed by what I'm going through with him that I honestly haven't given a rat's ass about anything else. I've been really self-destructive lately."

"Like how?" Lori asked.

"With booze and food. I was talking to my mom night last night, and once again, I've got her totally worried about me. She's 'done' with Rutherford at this point. She just wants me to get rid of him. She sees him as a big parasite. I don't understand why I do this crap to myself."

Lori sat quietly with the receiver in her hand. She let Angela continue to talk.

"I'm just feeling so *lost*. Really insecure. He's late all the time, hardly ever calls anymore … It hurts *so much*. It's like I'm just an 'after-thought' to him."

"Are you starting to doubt whether or not you love him?" Lori asked.

"No, it's more like I'm starting to doubt *his* love for *me*. I know I love the guy. I mean, I never really did get over him. But he's admitted that he would never have been the one to get in touch with me. He says he just didn't want to risk rejection ... But you know, I think he just 'moved on' with his life and made me a part of his past."

"Hang in there, Angela," Lori said.

"Do you know what he told me last night, over the phone? I asked him if he *really* loved me, and he said, 'I don't know if I even know what real love is.'"

"Guess that wasn't quite the answer you were expecting or hoping for?" Lori asked.

"Not at all," Angela said. "But at least he was honest. He went on to say that he *felt* very much in love with me, and attracted to me, and all that. But that his actions didn't always show that and he doesn't know why. Do *you* think he loves me, Lori?"

"I think it gets really tricky when people try to define love. I mean like, sometimes I wonder if I've ever

324

genuinely been 'in love' with anyone, according to the traditional definition of being 'in love.' There are times I feel like I might love Nick, but then I think about it more, and can't say for sure how I really feel."

"People do get into trouble when they base other peoples' love on their own personal definitions. I don't want to be so hell-bent on what I think Rutherford's love should 'look' like that I ignore the love he's actually showing," Angela said. "You make a lot of sense. Except the part about loving Nick! I think if you had actually started dating Nick- for real- your feelings would fade pretty quickly. I don't know about you, but someone can't turn me on unless they're intelligent and stimulating. Paul, I'm sure, is incomparably smarter than Nick. In fact, I'd wager a bet than most people are. I think you'd eventually get so bored that you wouldn't even be able to get excited about him physically. I also think part of the reason you got so attracted in the beginning was because something was lacking in your relationship with Paul. You needed a 'release' and Nick provided it."

"Yeah, well. There's some truth in what you're saying," Lori said. "But honestly, I have a problem labeling anyone as 'dumb.' I mean, I trained with Nick in Belchertown, and trust me- he's far from stupid. I just think he doesn't care enough to try."

"I guess what I meant to say was that he doesn't seem all that 'deep and sensitive,' you know what I mean? Maybe he's sensitive about *himself*, but how compassionate is he, really? Could you sit down and analyze, like, politics or religion or psychology with him? I used to try getting into deep stuff with him on the phone when we were working together, and I could only go so far. He just didn't seem to have much capacity for depth. Don't you agree?"

"Yeah."

"Look," Angela said. "I have 'loved' people who are just as vile, if not more so. I just know that when these 'creeps' were in my life, I didn't love or respect myself all that much. And I can't help but wonder if it's the same for you. If you were a lot more self-assured, would you really have time or energy for someone like Nick? You don't have to answer me... But you might want to think about that."

"I guess the answer's probably 'no.' But I just ... have so many mixed up feelings, *still*, when it comes to him. It's like, every minute of every day I just see everything as being so *finite.* Kind of pathetic, even. And it's not like it's anybody's fault. It's life. It's like we've all been tossed into this weird mix, and we've been left to make of it whatever we *think* we should be making of it. I see someone like Nick, and there's something about the way he tries to wall himself off. It's like, the more he pulls away, the more I want to reach out to him. The more I want to try to make things *better* for him, you know?"

"So you're *strangely* attracted to Nick. In a physical sense. And maybe otherwise. We'll just leave it at that."

"Okay. It's left," Lori said.

From Lori Solomon6697@yahoo.com
have a nice new years

From: NickWarren557@hotmail.com
u too hun

Lori would have settled for the quiet, affable coolness that seemed to be developing between her and Nick, coolness that was interrupted every so often by Nick's lusty volcanic upheavals printed out unabashedly in a stream of barely intelligible messages. She would have acclimated just fine, as the tides seemed to be turning in the direction of a light-hearted camaraderie only mildly tainted by the wanton remnants of their past.

But the tides turned again. Lori sent out messages that were met without any reply. She found herself battling the same recurring flurry of winged creatures in the pit of her stomach, the same shrinking of her heart as her ribcage wrapped itself tightly around it and pinched hard into its deflated ventricles. A seemingly perfect landing was suddenly met with gusty turbulence and she found herself hurled off-course to crash and burn.

"Why haven't you returned any of my messages?" she asked him, unable to control her irregular breathing into the phone receiver.

"Aah, I dunno. Just trying to drive you crazy," he replied, casually.

"Trying to drive me crazy?"

"Yeah." He laughed.

"What's going on?"

"Nothin'."

She remained quiet.

He remained quiet.

"I don't understand why you're being this way," she said. "What do you want to do? Where are we going now?"

"I dunno. Let's just let things go, see what happens."

She sighed into the phone. "Just two weeks ago, you were... I don't know. So... different toward me. You always leave this... question mark hanging over my head."

He grunted something unintelligible into the receiver.

"What do you want to do?" she repeated.

He shuffled the phone. "Let's just let things ride the way they have been."

"I can't," she said.

He paused. "All right."

"I don't think we should be in touch anymore," she said.

"Okay! If that's what you want!" he said, chuckling. "It's up to you."

"That's what I want," she said, before hanging up the phone.

From Lori Solomon6697@yahoo.com
i'd like to know what your problem is
i'd like to be friends with you, but i don't know if that's possible.
do you even know how to be friends with me with all that we've been through?

From: NickWarren557@hotmail.com
yeah, i know how to be friends.
but we've been friends "with benefits"
it makes it totally different
and sometimes totally annoying
like how many times in the past did you call me after i didn't return an e-mail of yours?

From Lori Solomon6697@yahoo.com
for some reason, you've been playing all these controlling little games with me
 and i have no idea why.

From: NickWarren557@hotmail.com
ok
i'm sorry if i bothered you.
look
you and i have our own lives.

i've really enjoyed those times we've had together,
but i've always tried not to get emotionally attached,
and i never wanted you to, either.
but obviously you did!
i've learned to walk away from things that are a problem.
i've learned not to get stressed over things that i can walk away from.
i think more people have to learn how to be that way.

From Lori Solomon6697@yahoo.com
being female it's hard not to get emotionally attached
i'm sorry, but when it comes to sex, that's just the way it is
and so…
i think at this point, i want more of a friendship with you than anything else.
i just think it'll work better in the long-run for both of us …

From: NickWarren557@hotmail.com
ok i guess we'll have to see
but if our friendship becomes a friendship with benefits …
try not to take it emotionally!

Asking her to twist her flesh around another's and then walk away as though she had just prepared a pitcher of unsweetened pink lemonade was like asking her not to blink or breathe. How could he make such a request? Knowing her the way she had allowed him to know her, how could he realistically have assumed that she would be the least bit successful in doing what obviously came so naturally to someone like him?

Just the same, asking him to view her only platonically and then treat her accordingly was undoubtedly just as absurd of a request. It had become both habitual as well as instinctual for both of them to claw feverishly at each other's loins when in each other's presence. It was all they knew of each other, and even if there was more to be discovered, anything beyond the carnal realm paled in comparison. At least it seemed to in Nick's mind.

There was soon a flurry of messages from Nick. Wormy bait delicately lowered into the freshwater pond, innocently bobbing up and down in tune with the easy current. She knew about the lure. Her lip was still swollen and bruised from the last time the hook had pierced it. And yet she still hungrily eyed the bait.

From: NickWarren557@hotmail.com
so any plans for tomorrow night?

From Lori Solomon6697@yahoo.com
no

From: NickWarren557@hotmail.com
would you wanna meet up and go out?

She envisioned parking her car behind his dusty Ford Thunderbird, and creeping along the length of the front lawn as she neared the side porch entrance. She could see the same fluffy white cat that had been there the last time watching her suspiciously as she quietly ascended the frail steps of the wooden deck. She could see Nick standing silently in the doorway under the dim porch light, peering at her with his head bent, expectantly.
She would walk inside, and step carefully down the narrow stairway to the basement. The floor mat saying,

"WELCOME," would have been kicked to one side, and she would walk past it toward the covered pool table. She would be standing awkwardly in the center of the room, playing with the buttons on her long-sleeved blouse, fumbling nervously with the contents of her purse. He would pull her near to him, and they would become one. They would belong to each other for a string of isolated moments, moments as separate as film frames, moments moving fast enough to give only the illusion of continuance.

And then they would become strangers, again.

From Lori Solomon6697@yahoo.com
i want to wish you a happy birthday
as a "gift," i'm giving you my friendship …
without benefits
i really can't do it anymore
but i still really do want us to be friends

From: NickWarren557@hotmail.com
hehe ok hunny!
thanks for the birthday greeting

i've learned to walk away from things that are a problem. i've learned not to get stressed over things that i can walk away from. Lori was filled with envy. She longed for the ability to just … walk away. And yet, she knew that dragging something on that she knew wasn't going anywhere- something that would most likely only end up perishing in a burst of flames the longer it was allowed to just continue- was worse than simply turning in the other direction. She supposed she was missing some kind of vital "survival" instinct, the one that would let her know when it was time to move on.

She knew deep down inside that she didn't have Nick, and she knew that she most likely would never have Nick. Yet the loss of what she knew she couldn't have would have been another heart-wrenching loss in a long series of losses. She wanted desperately to break the pattern of losing, even if it meant going very much against the odds. She wanted to attain the unattainable, for it was only the conquering of the unconquerable that would bring justice to Lori's past, itself unattainable and unconquerable in her eyes.

Chapter 30

Do not look where you fell, but where you slipped
African Proverb

From: AngelontheAirwaves3254@hotmail.com
Subject: Re:
To: LoriSolomon6697@yahoo.com
Well, Lori, Rutherford's gone. One argument and that was it. It's just beyond my comprehension that he could walk away from what we had without looking back even ONCE. It doesn't even seem human. I've just never been in a situation where a relationship has ended so abruptly with no reasonable discussions after the dust has settled. I would venture to get in touch with him, but everyone- and I mean EVERYONE- has told me that would be like nailing myself to a cross. I would be setting myself up for God knows what. And it would not be good. So, I'm keeping myself from contacting him by writing him countless letters that will never be sent. That bastard.
He said he knows I'm "better off" without him; that he always seemed to be doing or saying something to hurt me, and he was trying to "respect" my need to have him out of my life. But I don't buy it. I really just think he's too lazy to "fight" for me, or even apologize for how he wronged me. When a guy tells a girl "you're too good for me," that is classic bull for "I'm really not that into you, because I'm not willing to do whatever it takes to BECOME good enough for you."
Angela

From: LoriSolomon6697@yahoo.com
Subject: Re:
To: AngelontheAirwaves3254@hotmail.com

I guess sometimes with people, if you feel they're "slipping away," maybe it's best to just let go? It doesn't have to be forever- maybe just for a period of time until the dust settles. Maybe when you're feeling up to it you could talk to him, if you think the relationship means enough to you.
Lori

From: AngelontheAirwaves3254@hotmail.com
Subject: Re:
To: LoriSolomon6697@yahoo.com
Lori, I used to be JUST like you in that I wanted to "talk things out" ad nauseum with every bloody person in my life. I'm not like that anymore. I've gone through too much pain at the hands of supposedly caring friends and boyfriends to want to give anyone third and forth and fifth and infinitum chances. I read your letter and thought to myself, this is what Lori would do, but I'm not Lori and this is not what "the new self-affirming" Angela would do. I'm not going to get anywhere trying to talk to Rutherford- a person who has shown his "true colors" in that he can't take responsibility for his bad behaviors.
Angela

From: LoriSolomon6697@yahoo.com
Subject: Re:
To: AngelontheAirwaves3254@hotmail.com
Then I think you should just let go. Sometimes it's not worth it. I'm starting to find that out for myself with some of my own experiences with people. Life really doesn't have to be as complicated as some people insist on making it. It's up to us to simplify. I tend to give people the benefit of the doubt, probably more so than I should a lot of the time.
Lori

From: AngelontheAirwaves3254@hotmail.com
Subject: Re:
To: LoriSolomon6697@yahoo.com
I guess I'm feeling more and more like I should live by the rule "hurt me once, shame on you; hurt me twice, shame on me." And in both of our cases (you with Nick and me with Rutherford), we were hurt by them dozens of times. I think this goes beyond "giving someone the benefit of the doubt." It just makes us look like professional victims, rather than "wicked altruistic."
Every day I find myself remembering a way in which Rutherford took advantage of me, and I just "let it go." Or I remember times when I would be crying in pain, and he would be ice cold- showing no emotion, and then laughing hysterically about something thirty seconds later. There were so many things I went through with him that I never told you or anyone about because I wanted so much for that relationship to work out. Don't know why, I still can't figure it out, but that's what I wanted. And the fact that I haven't heard one word from him tells me all I need to know. He's probably moved on to some other "sucker" whom he can use for whatever he can get.
I'm writing this more for myself than you. I'm just now beginning to really understand Rutherford, and his M.O. What I need to explore more is WHY I let myself become one of his "victims."
Angela

From: LoriSolomon6697@yahoo.com
Subject: Re:
To: AngelontheAirwaves3254@hotmail.com
Angela,
I just think there's a fine line between doing that and beating yourself up over something that happened with someone whose behavior you had no control over. I

find myself sometimes late at night agonizing over why I allowed myself to get taunted one day in ninth grade gym class by a bully. I can't erase the fact that it DID happen, and that I ALLOWED it to happen. But how is it helping me now to revisit that experience over and over again, feeling every time the memory strikes like I'm still that shy awkward kid who was frozen like a deer in headlights? How is it helping me to have all that old anger welling up inside of me, part of it directed at the bully for causing it to happen, and part of it directed at myself for letting it happen? You can't reverse the past. You can only understand it as best you can to try to avoid the same problems in the future. But overanalyzing why someone did what they did and why you allowed them to do what they did is only going to make one person suffer long after the experience is over. And that's YOU.

Lori

Lori sat quietly on a pillow cushioning the rickety wooden chair in front of her computer. She thought about how close and intense relationships had the potential to be, and how amazing it was that such intimacy and intensity could be so easily replaced at the blink of an eye by abandon and distance. It was the emptiness within that could draw people together. It was the emptiness within that could split people apart.

"Finiteness." "Impermanence." Perhaps everything that happened in life-- the blink of love, the blink of sex, and the blink of life itself-- was just part of a larger continuum, as opposed to a tease or a taunt whose fate was inevitably to be mourned. Perhaps nothing in life really had to be thought of as meaningless so long as the heart and the mind were open to learning and growing. And nothing in life really had to die, so long as the heart and the mind were open to keeping it alive.

It would be possible, if it weren't for the stone slabs that Lori felt were slowly stacking around her heart, one on top of the other. Every time she felt she had lost trust, a stone was set and locked in place. Every time she felt she lost a friend, every time she felt she had lost herself, another stone was layered on top of the previous one, making it harder to keep an open mind and an open heart. She felt that she had been like a piece of bread that had been left in the toaster too long. The fringes had become blackened and charcoal-like, not wholly desirable although still edible. Life was charring her. Though she appeared hardened, in fact she crumbled quite easily.

She wanted desperately to matter. She wanted desperately to mean something. To someone. To anyone. But it was getting so hard to see past the stone slabs. They were piling up so high that she was squinting. She was straining. Her eyes were beginning to ache.

"Paul?"
"Hey, Lori! How's it goin'?"
She and Paul talked for a while, like the two old friends that they had become, like the two old friends that they still were. She felt an old familiar, soothing calm that she had not felt in some time. She held onto the receiver and stroked its rim, pretending it was Paul's cheek. His face had always been clean-shaven and full, not stubbly and concave like Nick's. If she thought hard about it, she realized that Paul's face was easier to caress than Nick's was... There was more for her to feel against the side of her hand when she swept it past his cheek. And she could do it without hesitation. She could do it without fear that she was getting too close, that he would pull away from her at any moment. And

Paul's eyes would always look deeply into her own as she did this, as opposed to Nick's, which were usually either closed or focused on something other than her. Although she had touched just about every stretch of furry skin on Nick's body, she had ironically never felt like anything less than a complete stranger to him.

She said good-bye and gently hung up the phone. She sat in her chair and stared peacefully at her computer screen. She wondered what it would be like to wake up in the morning and not be struck with a feeling of angst, not sure if that particular day would be another day of grim disappointment, or if it would be a miraculous turning point. She wondered what it would be like to travel down the middle of the road of life, instead of racing from one roadside ditch to another.

It would undoubtedly be different. But for someone like Lori, someone who harbored a soul so difficult to satiate, so difficult to satisfy, while it would be different, would it be better? If she were on the verge of plunging into a different kind of life, maybe a simpler kind of life, then what was the purpose of all that she had experienced up to then? Had it all been to guide her to something she otherwise wouldn't be able to find on her own and appreciate? Or was it all meant to sit in her memory as a constant reminder of who she really was, lest she try to forget?

She supposed it might be easier for her to propel forward if she were filled with regret, but all she could feel was a kind of perverse gratitude that she was able to experience what she had. Perhaps she was slipping into a phase of life that meant she would fair better without so much uncertainty, but it didn't mean that she wouldn't, on occasion, miss the uncertainty. For it was the uncertainty that made her journey both painful and interesting, evoking similar feelings to those her brother claimed he had when he worked all night in the laboratory only to get results the following morning that he couldn't interpret. It was a tough combination to find in life, as well as a tough combination to deal with once it was found. Yet it was a combination that was hard to forget, and with Nick, it was one that she would find herself thinking about for years to come.

A message appeared on Lori's computer. It was from Rutherford. She hadn't been hearing from Rutherford very often while he had been with Angela. During that time she had felt that he was on the verge of drifting out of her life for good, as though he could only handle one female confidante in his life at a time and having more than one would be like an admission on his part that females actually served a functional purpose on this planet other than to be scorned and demeaned.

From: SeriousSchmendrick4428@aol.com
Subject: Festering boil
To: LoriSolomon6697@yahoo.com
I can't really say that I've been "busy" in the true sense of the word. However, I've been undergoing some sort of character metamorphosis lately wherein I've been questioning every fiber of my ... um ... character. Was I a BAD person in years past? Did I do anything RIGHT? Was it all necessary in the process of positive personal evolution? Regardless, the changing has me wondering if I've historically perceived the world around me correctly and it has been causing a certain level of neurotic insecurity that results in me not having much to say, I think. I guess that's the best way to describe it.
Anyway, my new job is pretty cool, but I've been having a slightly difficult time forcing myself to hold my tongue when I feel like being a wise ass or ridiculing anyone in a position of authority over me. Something tells me that

if I learn to keep my mouth shut I'll do better in life than I've convinced myself previously.

I must to the bed. Whatever that means.

I shall speak to you expediently. Oh, by the way. If you run into a guy named Fortuna, don't speak to him. If you do, don't believe anything he might say about me. He's one of THEM.

Rutherford

Slowly moving her mouse across the length of its pad, she started clicking away old messages from Nick on her computer. She watched closely as each began to vanish with short taps on the mouse and keys, like smoking guns removed from the scene of a crime. After closing out of her e-mail site, her eyes fell on an instant messenger window, with the name "August West00001," bold-faced and active and beckoning for attention. August West00001 was Nick Warren's screen name. She clicked on the words twice, and watched as an instant messenger screen appeared with the blinking bar prompt ready to go.

Lori S what's up?
August West00001 nada
August West00001 u
Lori S nothing much
August West00001 so what u wearing … lol
Lori S sweat pants and an oversized t-shirt
August West00001 kool
August West00001 u miss it
Lori S i have to go
August West00001 hehe
August West00001 bye
August West00001 so why u leavin
August West00001 do i bother you
Lori S at times

Lori S i don't know
August West00001 i know i do
Lori S then why do you?
August West00001 i just do ... it's me
August West00001 u love me ... admit it
Lori S huh?
August West00001 never ond
August West00001 ond
August West00001 mond
August West00001 mind
August West00001 so what are your plans
August West00001 any pleasure involved in your day?
Lori S nah
Lori S you?
August West00001 yup
Lori S well, think of me! i guess
Lori S or someone
Lori S i don't know
Lori S forget i said that
August West00001 i do sometimes
August West00001 think of you when i do it
Lori S i'll talk to you again sometime

She signed out. Logging back on several minutes later, she saw that "August West00001" had turned a pale gray. It was idle now.

Chapter 31

Church ain't over until the fat lady sings
Southern Proverb

The days began to pass. And the days slipped into weeks. At the end of each week, Lori continued to write and voice biotechnology reports for the Belchertown business station. Paul usually accompanied her, waiting quietly and patiently among the cold, sterile cubicles outside the stuffy little production studio until she had finished her work. Weekend after weekend, this was the tireless routine, until the receipt of a terse e-mail from the station's general manager telling her that her services had fallen victim to a sweeping budget cut.

On rare occasions, she would receive a joke from a friend that she thought Nick would like, and she would send it to him. On even more rare occasions, he would acknowledge having received the joke, and he would ask her how she was doing. She would tell him she was well, and then she wouldn't hear from him again. Until the next joke that was sent that he felt like randomly acknowledging.

From: NickWarren557@hotmail.com
u know i don't work at buz anymore?

From: LoriSolomon6697@yahoo.com
i didn't know that ... what happened?

From: NickWarren557@hotmail.com
i'm doing something else now

From: LoriSolomon6697@yahoo.com
doing what?

From: NickWarren557@hotmail.com
i actually got a job building stonewalls. i'll get you some
pix of the work i did

So Nick was no longer involved in broadcasting
either. He was instead building stonewalls. According to
Mitch, Nick had been let go from the station, so that
someone new could be hired to take his place.
Jonathan had reputedly at long last bought the business
station. Yet shortly after its purchase, he was curiously
on the verge of selling it to another prospective buyer.
The incoming owner had been for months in the
process of revamping the station, and that included
letting go of certain old full-time staffers, like Nick, and
replacing them with new hires. Perhaps the new person
replacing Nick was someone believed to be more
capable than Nick. Perhaps the new person was
someone believed to be as capable as Nick, but willing
to do his job for far less money. And in broadcasting, it
seemed to only take a wink and a nudge and a referral
to poor station ratings to oust someone from any
position, no matter how dedicated the person, and often
... no matter how good or talented the person.
Lori felt as badly for Nick as she did for herself. At
the same time she was intrigued by the irony of his
being paid to do something now that for years he had
been in many ways paying a price for doing. If there
was anyone who believed with heartfelt conviction in
the importance of building impenetrable barriers, it was
Nick, and Lori was happy to see him slip so effortlessly
into a niche he seemed to be custom made for.

More days elapsed. More weeks. More jokes were
sent out. More indiscriminate replies were received.
How was someone like him still in the periphery of her
life? Was it simply her diligence that kept him there, or

was it something more? And why, after all this time, did Lori still care ... so damn much?

She e-mailed a joke to him that she had gotten from her uncle Hyman, and then stepped away from the computer to grab some buttered bread and a cup of hot cocoa. When she returned, munching and sipping, she noticed that Nick had sent an e-mail back to her.

From: NickWarren557@hotmail.com
you got your instant messenger on?

Lori's palms were clammy when his screen name appeared in bold on her computer, a yellow smiley face at its side. It felt like it had been such a long time.

August West00001 u want to play soon
August West00001 just got a cam in the mail for my puter ... its pretty cool
August West00001 u want to see
August West00001 let me know how the picture is

She watched as a new box appeared on her screen, asking her if she wanted to view Nick Warren's web cam. She clicked "yes," and waited. His face soon appeared, a little blurry, although noticeably unshaven and gaunt. His wild, curly dark hair was messily tucked under a baseball cap. His eyes looked tired, and his face seemed worn, as though roughened by a few too many taxing days and far too few serene nights.

She wondered if he was okay. She wondered if he was lonely. She wanted to reach out to him, touch him, and hold him in her arms. She wanted to sweep her hand over his forehead and rake his hair with her fingers.

August West00001 cute huh?

Lori S yes
August West00001 u want me
August West00001 i haven't had any in ages
Lori S why not?
August West00001 just no luck in getting any
Lori S sorry to hear that
August West00001 i almost forgot what it feels like to be with a female

The box that encased his frail-looking, haggard image turned black. Lori waited for a few seconds to see if his face would reappear. It didn't.

 Lori S you just faded to black
August West00001 that's weird
Lori S yeah, what's up with that?
August West00001 am i there now
Lori S you're a big black box on my computer screen
August West00001 u there
Lori S i'm here
August West00001 see me
Lori S no
August West00001 see anything now
Lori S no
August West00001 now

The solid black rectangle in the center of her screen was quickly replaced by a still picture of his naked torso. She could see the outline of his ribs. There wasn't a trace of fat around his middle. He definitely looked like he had lost weight since the last time she had seen him. He just looked like he had been through so much.

August West00001 u see
Lori S quite well, actually

345

August West00001 u like
Lori S you're gone again ... faded to black
Lori S you're back again
August West00001 turn u on ...
Lori S it's interesting ...
August West00001 u want more
Lori S sure
August West00001 wish i was there
August West00001 u want me
August West00001 u like this
Lori S yes

She leaned back in her chair and continued watching him. Occasionally he would position the camera so that it captured his jubilant face, which had a satisfied smile spanning from ear lobe to ear lobe. As he danced in front of the web cam, he typed messages to Lori.

August West00001 i could blindfold you
August West00001 and tie your hands to my bed posts

She waited for his words to seize her, and to make her slip into his world and dive headlong into the fantasy. She felt that it had been such a long time since they had related to one another in this way. Yet, upon seeing him after the passage of a very long span of time, her heart surprisingly seemed quieter, calmer than it used to be. She didn't feel an unnerving chill bound recklessly down her spine; she didn't have an aching that she had to squeeze her thighs together to suppress. She couldn't understand why she felt so far removed from everything that he was proposing, and why his words were bouncing off of her like she was enveloped in some kind of protective shield. She wondered if it was because, after having taken such a long hiatus, he had returned only to have it be about him. Lori felt that she could just as easily be a call girl that he was parading around in front of and making propositions to. There was nothing in his words or his actions to make Lori feel that it mattered in the slightest that she was who she was, and that she was there.

Lori S we've known each other for such a long time now
August West00001 damn long time
August West00001 so u want to come over
Lori S now?
August West00001 no, but soon
August West00001 i am a very sexual person ... i want it everyday, more than once a day ... im good at it
Lori S i know you are
August West00001 i like to make the moment feel good ... let the other person just let go
August West00001 just let yourself free for a few passionate hours with me

She removed her fingers from the keyboard and sat quietly, staring at the moving picture on her computer. He was still dancing, and still smiling. She knew he was enjoying himself, at least at the moment. And that made her happy. Yet she was still oddly removed, unexpectedly at ease. His actions were just actions. His words were just words. She wanted more of a connection.

Lori S do you think i'm beautiful?
August West00001 yes
Lori S really
August West00001 yes
August West00001 i would date u
August West00001 hopefully u wanted sex every day

Lori S you never told me this before
Lori S thank you for telling me that
August West00001 your welcome
August West00001 tell me what u would do to me now
Lori S put my arms around you
Lori S massage your back, your shoulders
Lori S make you feel loved
August West00001 and
Lori S i guess that wouldn't be enough?
August West00001 would u want sex with me
August West00001 everyday
August West00001 with me
Lori S ummm
August West00001 tell me
August West00001 hey my cam died
Lori S hope that didn't destroy the moment for you
August West00001 errr
August West00001 it did
Lori S oh no
Lori S after all that work
August West00001 i know
August West00001 well go to bed
Lori S okay, have a nice night, Nick
August West00001 u 2
Lori S it's been fun ...

Lori stared at the computer screen. She watched August West00001 fade from black and bold to a pale gray. She left her computer on, crawled onto her nearby bed and slipped under a plush comforter. The radiator sitting under her drafty bedroom window hissed and sputtered, trying to cut through the cool air circulating in the room. Lori wriggled underneath her bedcovers, and began to feel the discomfort of the chilly night ease as she basked in the quirky warmth of knowing that Nick had become a mere click away from contact. Once again.

The days passed, as well as the nights. And the days became perched and ready to turn into weeks. August West00001 was unyieldingly pale and gray and idle in the far right-hand corner of her computer screen. Had he suddenly become unbearably busy? Was he traveling? Was he in some kind of trouble? Or was he actually silently and sneakily there, in "invisible mode," spying on Lori every time she logged onto her instant messenger account at different times of the day, and waiting for that perfect moment to pounce back into her life like a jaguar after just enough time had drifted by to mount the tension, and to make Lori want him all the more desperately. To make him want her.

It was a brisk winter morning, and it seemed much like any other brisk winter morning until Lori scanned the front page of one of the local newspapers and saw something that made any of her concerns over Nick seem ridiculously inconsequential. "Ripped-off investors..." "Con artist..." "Subtle scheme..." "Mail fraud..." "Dramatic confession..." "Wife unaware..." "Freezing of Mogul's Assets..." "Prospective buyer pulls out..." "Scandal..." "Deceit..." "Tragedy..."

Lori's eyes couldn't take in all the information fast enough. Line after line in the front-page article described station owner Jonathan's mimicking of a scam based on that of Charles Ponzi, who, back in 1920, swindled 10 million dollars in six month's time from trusting investors. Jonathan had apparently stolen millions of dollars from clients of his firm over a span of decades, and had used at least some of the stolen money to purchase WBUZ. He had gotten caught. And now he was going to jail.

Ponzi scheme. Deception. Lori couldn't believe it. She *knew* this person. She knew this person as seemingly friendly, confident, successful. How could this be? Suddenly, he was spotlighted as having led a life of deception, a life with a heavy payoff for the short-term, followed by a heavy cost for the long-term. Why did he choose this for himself? Wouldn't it have been better to have led a life of quiet calm- no thrills, no chills, but with no pretense? Wouldn't it have been better to have lived with nothing to hide, and nothing in the end to regret?

Lori listened to the sounds of heavy breathing coming from the next room. It was Paul, sleeping in on that brisk winter morning while Lori read about Jonathan in the newspaper. It was gentle Paul, slumbering away in Lori's twisted sheets, under her soft, plush comforter. Quiet calm. No pretense, nothing to hide, and nothing in the end to regret.

Lori positioned her mouse so that with a couple of clicks August West00001, pale and gray and seemingly idle, disappeared. Again. A sharp-shooting pain swept through her insides as she stared at the computer screen. She drew a deep breath and let the air very slowly out of her lungs. She knew it was the right thing to do, regardless of the feeling in her gut.

From: NickWarren557@hotmail.com
sorry i haven't written in a while
been in the hospital
something's not working right
i'm home now
call me

What was this? An e-mail. He had contacted her. He had contacted *her*. He seemed to want to share something with her. He seemed to want to share something with *her*. *Share* something. With *her*.

"Are you okay?" Lori asked with heaviness in her voice she couldn't suppress. "What happened?"

"I don't wanna talk about it," he said. Silence followed.

"Can I visit you?" she asked.

"Sure. I'll give you the directions."

He had led her to a different place than she had been to in the past. It was a small house that he was renting with a roommate, and it was in a quiet neighborhood. She pressed down on a semi-lit doorbell and could soon hear him calling to her from a room inside.

He was kneeling on a couch in his living room when she entered. He looked small to her, like a little boy, with his thin, fragile legs bent under him and his nimble fingers wrapped around a television remote control. He paused the sporting event that was playing on his big screen TV and looked up at her.

"How are ya?" he asked.

"Fine," she said.

"Thanks for comin' here. I can show you around if you want."

"Sure."

He stood up and, waving his arms around, said, "This is our living room." He took a few steps toward the back of the house. "This is the bathroom, in case you have to *go*. Here's my roommate's room, here's my room. Here's our kitchen…"

"Nice little place you guys have here," Lori said. She noticed a stuffed animal sitting by Nick's bedside. She felt a jolt of envy looking at it. She thought about someone giving him something that he felt strongly enough about to keep, and display.

"Do you wanna cuddle with me in my room?" he asked.

"Yes."

They lay down together on his bed. She rested her head on his shoulder, and he placed his arm around her and caressed the small of her back with his hand. She swept her hand gently back and forth across his chest, causing him to moan softly with each stroke. She slipped her fingers underneath his shirt and massaged his bare skin.

"It's been such a long time since I've been with a woman," he said. "I've practically forgotten what it feels like."

She continued to caress his skin, and he continued to moan. She felt like they could lie like that forever, next to each other, cuddling. Just being together. It was the first time she had ever been with him in which just being close to one another seemed to be enough.

She leaned her head closer to his. He turned his face toward her and kissed her softly on her mouth. He gently pulled her hand from where it rested on his stomach and placed it over his chest so she could feel his heart thumping.

"See? It's working *now*," he said, chuckling.

Lori could hear rain pouring outside the wall of his bedroom. It sounded like torrents were gushing from the roof and smacking hard against the ground. She pictured the world outside weeping uncontrollably as she and Nick drew closer and relived their past one last time. The rainwater continued to beat fiercely into the ground. Nick would be gone just a few months later.

Knowing Nick made Lori look at her life differently. Knowing him made Lori look at life itself differently.

Perhaps it was enough for her to know that, at the very least, she made a ripple in his still deep pond, cold as fresh fallen rainwater after an autumn storm. Nick wanted her, as much as he could want anyone who was so different from him. She wanted him, more than anything because he was so different from her. And she knew that in ways that stemmed beyond just the physical, they had touched each other, and not in spite of their differences, but *because* of their differences.

If she ever did eventually walk down the aisle, she knew a part of her would linger behind, unable to take those steps, unable to take any vows. And that part of her was the part that Nick would always have. It was the part of her that was so filled with emptiness, there just wasn't enough there for her to give to anyone she was able to physically or emotionally feel, hear, or even see. It was a part of her that was equivalent to the part of Nick that he had allowed her to have: an illuminated type-written name boxed into a corner of her computer screen.

"I am going to put you in my book some day," she remembered Nick seductively boasting to her early on in their affair, despite the fact that there probably wasn't an editor alive at the time with the proper balance of patience and allegiance to work with him. And years later, long after he was gone, Lori would find herself walking into a bookstore, looking for her name on a shelf, and his name on a page.